UNRAVELLING THE MYSTERY OF IMMUNOLOGY: HOW OUR IMMUNE SYSTEM RECALLS PAST EVENTS TO PROTECT US TODAY

D. Beck

Cover design by: Art Painter
Library of Congress Control Number: 2018675309
Printed in the United States of America

I Want to thank you and congratulate you for buying my book
Unravelling the Mystery of Immunology

CONTENTS

INTRODUCTION

The immune system is a complex network of cells, tissues and organs that protect the body from infection. It helps to identify and destroy bacteria, viruses, and other pathogens that can cause disease. The immune system also plays an important role in fighting off cancer cells and other abnormal cells. The different components of the immune system work together to recognize, attack, and eliminate harmful substances.

The primary components of an immune system are the white blood cells, also known as leukocytes. These cells travel throughout the body looking for foreign substances that may be harmful to the body. The lymphatic system is a network of organs and tissues that collect and store these cells so they can quickly respond to any potential threats. Additionally, the spleen helps filter out bacteria and other particles, while the thymus helps train immature white blood cells to become mature.

The immune system also relies heavily on the production of antibodies. Antibodies are special proteins that recognize and bind to specific foreign substances in the body. Once an antibody binds to a substance, it triggers an immune response which can be either localized or systemic depending on the type of pathogen and the size of its attack.

The immune system also depends heavily on communication between cells. Cells communicate with each other through a variety of methods, including cytokines, chemokines, interferons, and many other molecules. Each type of cell has different receptors for these signals, allowing them to respond appropriately to different threats.

The immune system is an incredibly complex and remarkable network of cells, tissues, and organs that work together to protect the body from infection. Without the immune system, our bodies would be vulnerable to many different forms of disease. Taking good care of your immune system is a key part of maintaining overall health and wellness. Eating a balanced diet, getting regular exercise, and managing stress levels can all help to keep your immune system performing at its best

Hello, it's me, D.Beck . Before you start reading my book I would like to ask you a favor: If you enjoy reading the book can you please leave an honest review for me in Amazon? - it will mean a lot to me! Thanks in advantage, and now be ready to learn how to understand your immune system :)

CHAPTER 1: IMMUNE SYSTEM

T he immune system is a complex network of cells, tissues, and organs that works together to protect your body from harmful agents such as bacteria, viruses, fungi, and parasites. It helps defend against disease-causing microorganisms by identifying and destroying these invaders while also keeping an eye out for any abnormal changes in the body's own cells. The immune system is essential for protecting us from illness, and it continues to develop and adapt throughout our lifetime.

Basics Immunity

The body's immune system is a complex and dynamic network of cells, tissues, and organs that protect us against infection and disease. The immune system has two primary components: the innate immune system and the adaptive immune system. The innate immune system is comprised of physical barriers like skin, as well as chemical messengers such as cytokines that defend our bodies from bacteria and other invaders. The adaptive immune system, on the other hand, is made up of specialized cells that are able to recognize and respond quickly to specific threats.

Defense Against Infections

Defense against infections refers to the body's ability to recognize and respond quickly to certain threats, such as bacteria or viruses. The immune system is able to identify these foreign agents, then produce antibodies that can destroy them. This process helps protect us from diseases, illnesses, and other harmful organisms. Additionally, our bodies are equipped with a variety of mechanisms – such as white blood cells, mucous membranes, and skin – that work to prevent infections from entering the body. These mechanisms can also trigger inflammation in response to an infection, which helps protect our bodies from further damage. In short, our immune systems are constantly working to keep us healthy and safe from harm.

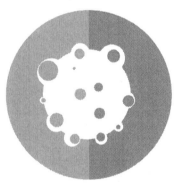

Defense Against Tumors

In addition to defense against infections, the immune system also plays an important role in defending us against tumors and other forms of cancer. Our bodies contain a variety of specialized cells that can detect when there is abnormal cell growth, then work to eliminate these cells in order to prevent them from growing into a tumor or cancerous mass. These specialized cells are known as natural killer cells, and they are an important component of our immune system.

Control Of Tissue Regeneration And Scarring

The immune system is also responsible for controlling tissue regeneration and scarring. After an injury or illness, our bodies undergo a process of healing in which the damaged cells are replaced with new ones. The immune system helps to control this process by recognizing when tissues are being regenerated and ensuring that they are properly replaced. Additionally, the immune system can help to minimize scarring by producing proteins that help promote healthy tissue regeneration.

Regulation Of The Body's Environment

The immune system is responsible for regulating our bodies' internal environments. This includes controlling the temperature, pH balance, and levels of electrolytes such as sodium and potassium in various parts of the body. By maintaining these levels within a normal range, the immune system helps to ensure that our bodies remain healthy and free from disease.

The Immune System Can Injure Cells And Induce Pathologic Inflammation

Though the immune system has many protective functions, it is also capable of harming cells and inducing inflammation. In some cases, the immune system can become overactive or misdirected, leading to an autoimmune attack on healthy cells. This often leads to a range of pathologic conditions that involve abnormal inflammation and tissue damage. It is important to understand that this type of response occurs when the immune system is functioning abnormally, and that it can be managed with proper medical treatment.

The Immune System Recognizes And Responds To Tissue Grafts And Newly Introduced Proteins

Finally, the immune system is able to recognize and respond to tissue grafts and newly introduced proteins. For example, when a transplanted organ or tissue is introduced into the body, the immune system will work to identify it as foreign. The body then produces antibodies that attack the new cells in order to protect against any potential risk they may pose. Similarly, when foreign proteins, such as those found in certain foods or medications, are introduced into the body, the immune system will produce antibodies in order to neutralize them. In this way, our bodies can recognize and respond to potential threats in order to keep us healthy.

How Does The Immune System Works ?

The immune system is the body's defense against infections and other foreign invaders. This complex network of cells, tissues, and organs helps to defend against bacteria, viruses, toxins, and parasites that may cause diseases. The immune system works in several ways to battle infection: it identifies pathogens; produces special antibodies and white blood cells; releases chemicals into the bloodstream to fight infection; and creates memory cells to recognize pathogens for future attacks.

The immune system also has the ability to distinguish between normal, healthy cells and foreign invaders. When a pathogen is detected, the immune system triggers an attack and activates specialized cells called lymphocytes. These lymphocytes produce antibodies that bind with the invading antigen, which marks it for destruction by other immune system cells. The cells also alert other parts of the body to start producing more antibodies so that they can continue attacking the antigen until it is destroyed.

How Does The Immune System Distinguish Among Pathogens ?

The immune system is a complex network of cells, tissues and organs that work together to protect the body from foreign invaders. These foreign antigens can come in many forms, including viruses, bacteria, fungi and parasites. When exposed to these invader organisms, the immune system responds with an array of defense mechanisms designed to eliminate the threat. One way it accomplishes this is by distinguishing between different types of pathogens.

The body has several mechanisms for making

this distinction, including the ability to recognize antigens that are specific to particular types of invaders. For example, when a virus enters the body, specialized cells called B cells recognize and bind to protein fragments on its surface, known as viral antigens. The binding triggers the activation of B cells, which then release antibodies that can target and neutralize the virus. On the other hand, when a bacteria enters the body, it has its own set of antigens on its surface, called bacterial antigens. These are recognized by different types of immune cells—specifically T cells and macrophages—which also activate to fight off the invader.

In addition to recognizing specific antigens, the immune system is also able to distinguish between types of pathogens based on their pathogenicity, or ability to cause disease. It does this by assessing the structure and function of the invading organism in order to determine if it poses a threat. For instance, some bacteria may be highly infectious but not particularly harmful, while others may cause severe disease. In these cases, the body can activate different defense mechanisms based on the pathogen's ability to cause harm.

The immune system is also able to recognize self from non-self antigens. This is an important distinction because if the body were unable to make this distinction, it could mistakenly attack its own cells and tissues, leading to autoimmune diseases. To prevent this from happening, the immune system has developed specialized receptors that are able to recognize antigens that belong to the body's own cells. This allows it to ignore or even destroy invading foreign antigens while leaving healthy tissue unharmed.

The ability of the immune system to distinguish between different types of pathogens and recognize self from non-self antigens is critical for protecting the body from disease. Through this complex process, it is able to quickly identify and eliminate threats while leaving healthy cells and tissues unharmed. This allows the body to effectively defend itself against a wide range of pathogens, including viruses, bacteria, fungi and parasites.

How Can The Immune System Recognise Different Germs ?

The immune system is incredibly complex and sophisticated, capable of recognizing and fighting off a vast number of different germs. It does this by using white blood cells that have molecular "receptors" on their surface. These receptors are designed to recognize specific molecules which can only be found on the surfaces of pathogens like bacteria or viruses. When these receptors recognize a pathogen, it triggers an immune response that leads to the production of more white blood cells and antibodies designed to fight off the infection.

In order to recognize a greater variety of pathogens, the body produces millions of different types of these receptors. Each type is designed to detect a specific molecular structure, meaning they can identify many different germs even if they look or behave differently from one another.

Once the immune system has recognized a pathogen, it will then begin producing antibodies that are specifically designed for attacking and neutralizing that particular germ. This process is known as "immunity" and is responsible for preventing us from getting sick or re-infected with the same disease.

It's important to note that even though the immune system is capable of recognizing and fighting off a wide variety of germs, it isn't always successful. Some pathogens are able to evade detection or even use our own bodies as a form of camouflage, meaning that they can avoid being destroyed by the immune system. If these types of germs spread unchecked, they can cause serious illnesses such as bacterial pneumonia and viral hepatitis.

Fortunately, there are vaccines available that can help the body to recognize and fight off certain pathogens without having to experience an infection first. Vaccines contain some form of the pathogen, either dead or weakened, and allow the immune system to develop a natural immunity against it before it has a chance to cause any harm. By vaccinating yourself against common diseases, you can ensure that your body is better equipped to fight off the germs that cause them.

Where In Your Body Is The Immune System?

The immune system is located throughout our body, from the skin barrier to the innermost organs. Our skin and mucous membranes form a physical barrier that prevents microorganisms from entering our bodies. The lymphatic system contains white blood cells – called lymphocytes – that are part of our adaptive immune system. This type of immunity is specific to each person and can recognize and remember different types of foreign invaders. The lymphatic system is also responsible for transporting pathogens from the body to be destroyed by the immune cells. Finally, our organs – such as the bone marrow, thymus, and spleen – house a variety of immune cells that provide protection against infections and diseases. Together, these structures comprise the complex immune system that helps keep us healthy.

So, while the immune system is generally thought of as a single functioning entity, it's actually composed of many different components that each play an important role in keeping us healthy. By understanding how our body's immune system works and where its various components are located, we can better protect ourselves from illness and disease. For example, good hygiene habits like regularly washing our hands and avoiding large crowds can help reduce our risk of contracting infectious diseases. Eating a healthy diet, getting enough rest, and exercising regularly are also important measures that can strengthen the body's immune system.

CHAPTER 2: COMPONENTS AND FUNCTIONS OF THE IMMUNE SYSTEM

T he immune system is composed of several components that work together to protect the body from pathogens and other foreign substances. One of the primary components of the immune system is B-cells, which produce antibodies that can bind to and neutralize invading antigens. T-cells are another important component; they recognize and eliminate infected cells by producing cytokines, which trigger an inflammatory response. Additionally, macrophages are specialized cells that can ingest and digest foreign particles that enter the body.

Components And Functions Of Lymphoid Organs

The lymphoid organs are a key component of the immune system, as they create and store white blood cells that help to fight off infection and disease. The main lymphoid organs include the thymus, spleen, tonsils, adenoids, Peyer's patches, and bone marrow.

Thymus

The thymus is a lymphoid organ located in the upper chest behind the sternum. It's comprised of two lobes, and it plays an integral role in the development and functioning of our immune system. The thymus helps to differentiate between

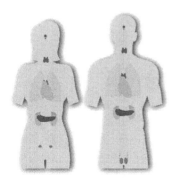

self and non-self molecules. Cells known as "T-cells" develop in the thymus and are responsible for recognizing foreign molecules from the body.

The thymus is most active during childhood and adolescence, when it helps to educate T-cells in the art of distinguishing between foreign antigens and our own molecules. It also serves as a site for T-cell maturation, providing an environment where these cells can learn how to respond to certain antigens. During this process, the thymus helps cells to become either "effector" or "memory" T-cells.

Effector T-cells are specialized in attacking foreign pathogens quickly and efficiently. Memory T-cells, on the other hand, are responsible for producing a rapid response against any pathogens that the body has already been exposed to. Both of these types of cells are essential for keeping us healthy and safe from infection.

As we age, the thymus begins to shrink in size and becomes less active. Unfortunately, this can lead to a weaker immune system, which is why it's important to look after our health throughout life in order to maintain a strong and functioning immune system.

Spleen

The spleen is a vital part of the human immune system, and plays an essential role in filtering blood, storing red blood cells, and producing certain types of white blood cells. It can also act as an immune system reservoir for ready-made antibodies which are released when needed to fight infection. The spleen is located in the upper left side of your abdominal cavity and consists of two types of tissue: red pulp and white pulp.

Red Pulp

The red pulp of the spleen is made up of small vascular sinuses that are lined with cells called macrophages. These macrophages filter the blood and remove unwanted debris, such as old or damaged red blood cells, from circulation. The red pulp also contains white blood cells which can rapidly respond to invading pathogens.

White Pulp

The white pulp of the spleen is made up of lymphocytes and macrophages that are responsible for producing antibodies and anti-viral compounds known as interferon. These antibodies can be released into circulation when needed to fight infection. The white pulp also contains small numbers of specialized cells called plasma cells which produce large amounts of specific antibodies against certain pathogens.

The spleen is important in helping the immune system recognize foreign pathogens, such as bacteria or viruses, and it also helps initiate an immune response to these threats. This organ can also help remove old or damaged red blood cells from the circulation and can store platelets for use in cases of extreme bleeding. Its role in the immune system makes it essential for proper functioning of the body's defense against disease.

Tonsils

Tonsils are part of the immune system that form a barrier at the back of the throat. They serve to trap bacteria and other pathogens traveling through the air or entering our body via food and water, alerting the immune system to their presence and prompting it to mount an attack against them. The tonsils act as a filtering mechanism, helping to protect us from infection. While tonsils are an important part of our immune system, they can also become infected and swollen due to a buildup of bacteria or viruses, which is known as tonsillitis. Symptoms of this condition include pain in the throat, difficulty swallowing, fever and bad breath. In some cases, antibiotics may be necessary to treat the infection; however, it is often possible to reduce the inflammation and clear the infection with home remedies and natural methods. These include drinking plenty of fluids, gargling salt water, taking probiotics and using essential oils. If these measures do not help then medical intervention may be needed to remove the tonsils or perform a tonsillectomy.

Over time, the tonsils can become enlarged and lead to more serious problems such as sleep apnea or difficulty breathing. In this case, medical treatment may be required to reduce the size of the tonsils and improve symptoms. Additionally, an infection in the tonsil area can spread to other parts of the body if not properly treated, making it important to get prompt medical attention if tonsillitis symptoms are present. By understanding the role of tonsils in our immune system and taking steps to protect them from infection, we can help ensure our bodies remain healthy and strong for years to come.

Bone Marrow

Bone marrow is an essential part of the immune system as it is where new white blood cells, or lymphocytes, are produced. The bone marrow also acts as a reservoir for B and T-cell precursors, which are types of lymphocytes that fight off pathogens. When the body senses danger from a foreign pathogen or virus, these precursors leave the bone marrow and enter circulation, where they can then identify and destroy any foreign invaders. Bone marrow is especially important in infants and young children as it helps to establish a strong immune system from an early age.

Bone marrow not only produces necessary

lymphocytes for immunity but also contains stem cells that are capable of generating new blood cells. These stem cells have been used in regenerative medicine to treat a variety of conditions, including leukemia, myeloma, and other blood-related disorders. Additionally, bone marrow contains macrophages and monocytes, which are types of white blood cells that specialize in phagocytosis (the ingestion and destruction of pathogens).

Peyer's Patches

Peyer's patches are specialized components of the intestinal immune system located in the lumen and walls of the small intestine. They play a critical role in defense against pathogens that enter through the intestines. The patches are made up of organized clusters of lymphoid follicles, which contain many different types of immune cells like B-cells, which secrete antibodies to fight infection, and macrophages, which can ingest foreign particles.

The primary function of the Peyer's patches is to act as a filter for the intestines. They have large numbers of specialized immune cells that can detect and eliminate potentially dangerous bacteria and other pathogens before they reach the rest of the body. In addition to acting as an effective barrier against infection, Peyer's patches also play an important role in the development and maintenance of a healthy immune system. They are essential for the proper functioning of the mucosal immune system, which is vital for protecting against infectious agents.

Peyer's patches are highly organized structures that can detect foreign antigens, activate local lymphocytes, and mount an effective response to pathogens. They are also involved in the digestion of dietary antigens, which can be beneficial for maintaining a balanced immune system. As such, Peyer's patches are an important part of the body's natural defense against infection and disease.

By providing essential protection against dangerous pathogens, Peyer's patches help to keep us healthy and safe from infection. It's important to maintain a healthy immune system to ensure that these patches are functioning properly. Eating a balanced diet, getting enough exercise, and getting regular checkups can all help keep Peyer's patches working effectively.

The Adenoids

The adenoids are an important part of the immune system. Located between the back of the nose and throat, they act as a filter for germs entering the body through the air we breathe. They produce antibodies that help fight off bacteria, viruses, fungi and other pathogens that can cause illness. In addition to their role in providing immunity, they also play a role in providing us with a healthy voice. The adenoids help to shape the sound of our speech and may even contribute to proper digestion by trapping food particles that could otherwise enter the stomach.

Adenoid problems, also known as adenoidal hypertrophy, can occur if they become enlarged due to allergies or infection. This condition can lead to difficulty breathing, snoring and sleep apnea. In severe cases, surgery may be required to remove the enlarged adenoids.

Adenoid problems can also occur in children due to frequent ear infections or allergies. If left untreated, adenoid hypertrophy can cause hearing loss as well as speech and language delays in children. Therefore it is important to seek medical advice if your child is experiencing these symptoms.

To prevent adenoid problems, it is important to maintain a healthy lifestyle and ensure you get enough rest each night. Avoiding allergens and irritants, such as smoke or strong odors, can also help keep the adenoids from becoming enlarged. Regular cleaning of the nose using a saline solution can help remove potential allergens and pathogens. Eating a healthy diet with plenty of fruits, vegetables, vitamins and minerals can also help keep the immune system strong, allowing it to fight off any foreign substances that may enter the body.

Lymph Nodes

Lymph nodes are small bean-shaped structures

that function as filters for the lymphatic system. They play an important role in helping to fight off diseases and infections by trapping viruses, bacteria, and other foreign particles. These particles are then broken down by white blood cells called macrophages, which can help the body to create antibodies against these invaders. Lymph nodes also contain specialized B cells and T cells —two essential types of white blood cell—that help the body to recognize and attack foreign invaders. Additionally, lymph nodes also produce cytokines, which are molecules that can stimulate other parts of the immune system in order to fight off infections. Finally, they act as processing centers for antigens—substances which trigger an immune response—and can help to produce and store antibodies.

Mucous Membranes

Mucous membranes, or mucosa, are the first line of defense for our immune system. They form a protective layer that covers the linings of organs and other body cavities. The mucosal surfaces act as a barrier to help keep out potentially harmful bacteria and viruses. These surfaces also house special cells called M-cells which can detect foreign materials and trigger an immune response. In addition, the mucosa produces mucus, a protective substance that helps trap and remove potentially dangerous particles before they can reach deeper tissues in our body.

The maintenance of healthy mucosal surfaces is critical for a strong immune system, which is why it's important to practice good hygiene habits like frequent hand washing and keeping up with regular health check-ups. Eating a balanced diet, getting enough sleep, and managing stress levels can also help keep our mucosal surfaces healthy and better able to protect us from invading pathogens.

Mucous membranes are key components of the immune system that serve many important functions in helping maintain our overall health and wellbeing. By taking care of these surfaces, we can ensure that our bodies are better prepared to fight off any invading microorganisms.

Immune Cells And Their Products

Interferon

Interferon is a type of protein that plays an important role in the body's immune system. It helps to protect cells from viral and bacterial infections. Interferon works by blocking viruses from entering into cells, thus preventing them from replicating and causing further damage. It also stimulates other parts of the immune system, such as activating white blood cells and increasing production of other proteins that help fight against invaders. Additionally, interferon can help reduce inflammation, which is often associated with autoimmune diseases. Interferon has been used for many years to treat a variety of conditions including viral infections, cancer, and autoimmune diseases such as multiple sclerosis. Scientists are continuing to research how interferon can be used in combination with other treatments for more effective results.

Interferon is a powerful tool in the body's fight against foreign invaders, and it has been instrumental in the development of many medical treatments. It is important to understand how interferon works so that we can continue to develop better treatments for diseases. As researchers learn more about interferon and its role in protecting cells from infection, they can develop new treatments and therapies to help improve the lives of people living with autoimmune diseases and other conditions. Interferon is an important component of a healthy immune system, and its role in defending against disease should not be underestimated.

Chemical Mechanisms Of Interferon

Interferon has several chemical mechanisms that help protect the body from infection. One main mechanism is to activate certain proteins in infected cells, such as interferon-stimulated gene products (ISGs). These proteins then interfere with viral replication, which helps stop the spread of the virus. Another important role of interferon is to stimulate the production of natural killer cells, which are immune system cells that can recognize and attack virus-infected cells. Interferon also stimulates the production of cytokines, which are small proteins that help regulate the immune response. Additionally, interferon can induce apoptosis, or programmed cell death, in infected cells so they cannot spread further infection.

Physical Mechanisms Of Interferon

Interferon also has physical mechanisms that can help protect the body from infection. One way it does this is by binding to receptors on the surface of cells, which triggers a response in the cell and helps stop viruses from entering into them. Interferon can also induce structural changes that make it harder for viruses to penetrate the cell membrane, thus preventing infection. Finally, interferon can stimulate the production of proteins that block viral replication and interfere with their life cycle.

These physical and chemical mechanisms work together to create an effective barrier against infection, helping the body fight off invaders and keeping us healthy. Interferon is a powerful part of the immune system, and its role in protecting us should not be underestimated.

Antibodies

Antibodies are proteins that help the immune system recognize and fight off foreign invaders such as bacteria and viruses. Antibodies are produced by B cells, which are a type of white blood cell. They work by binding to antigens on the surface of invading organisms, thus preventing them from entering into cells and causing infection. Once an antibody has bound to an antigen, it initiates a cascade of events that leads to the destruction of the invader.

Antibodies play an important role in protecting us from infection and disease. They are highly specific to their target antigens, meaning they can recognize and destroy just one type of organism at a time. This specificity allows antibodies to be effective against even highly mutated viruses or bacteria that might have changed in structure, allowing them to evade the immune system.

Antibodies are an important part of the body's natural defense system and help keep us healthy and safe from foreign invaders. They work in conjunction with other components of the immune system, such as interferon, to protect us from infection. By understanding how antibodies work and how they interact with other components of the immune system, we can develop better treatments and therapies to fight disease and keep us healthy.

Chemical Mechanisms Of Antibodies

Antibodies work in several ways to fight infection. First, they recognize and bind to antigens on the surface of invading organisms. This binding triggers a cascade of events that leads to the destruction of the invader. Additionally, antibodies can activate other parts of the immune system such as complement proteins and natural killer cells, which further help protect against infection.

Another important role of antibodies is to neutralize toxins that are produced by bacteria and other invaders. They do this by binding to the toxin and inactivating it, thus preventing it from causing damage to cells. Finally, antibodies can also help mark foreign organisms for recognition and destruction by other components of the immune system such as phagocytes.

Physical Mechanisms Of Antibodies

Antibodies also have physical mechanisms that help protect the body from infection. One of these is to recognize and bind to antigens on the surface of foreign organisms. This binding triggers an immune response, which helps fight off the invader. Additionally, antibodies can help block toxins produced by bacteria, thus preventing them from causing damage to cells. Finally, antibodies can also mark foreign organisms for recognition and destruction by other components of the immune system such as phagocytes.

Cytokines

Cytokines are small proteins that help regulate

the immune system and play an important role in fighting infections. Cytokines can be secreted by a variety of cells, including macrophages, B cells, and T cells. They help to regulate the body's response to infection by activating or suppressing certain parts of the immune system. For example, cytokines can stimulate the production of antibodies or activate natural killer cells, which help destroy infected cells.

Cytokines also play an important role in triggering inflammation, which is a necessary part of wound healing and recovery from infection. By understanding how cytokines work and how they interact with other components of the immune system, researchers can develop new treatments and therapies to improve the body's response to infection.

Chemical Mechanisms Of Cytokines

Cytokines work in several ways to help the body fight off infection. When cytokines are secreted by immune cells, they bind to receptors on other cells and trigger an immune response. This helps activate certain parts of the immune system such as B cells and natural killer cells, which can then attack foreign invaders. Cytokines also stimulate the production of inflammatory molecules, which helps to fight off infection and repair damage caused by invading organisms.

Additionally, cytokines also play an important role

in the activation of T cells, which are a type of white blood cell that can recognize specific antigens on the surface of foreign invaders. Once activated, T cells can help mark infected cells for destruction or release chemicals that can kill viruses or bacteria.

Finally, cytokines can also interact with certain hormones in the body such as cortisol and adrenaline to help regulate the immune response. By understanding how these hormones work together with cytokines, researchers can develop better treatments and therapies to fight infection.

Physical Mechanisms Of Cytokines

In addition to their chemical mechanisms, cytokines also have physical mechanisms that help fight infection. For example, they can bind to receptors on the surface of other cells and activate them. This helps stimulate an immune response and activate certain components of the immune system such as T cells or natural killer cells. Additionally, cytokines can also help mark foreign organisms for destruction by other components of the immune system such as phagocytes.

Cytokines also help regulate inflammation by triggering the production of molecules that are involved in wound healing and recovery from infection. Finally, cytokines can interact with hormones such as cortisol and adrenaline to help modulate the body's response to infection.

By understanding how these hormones work together with cytokines, researchers can develop better treatments and therapies to fight infection.

Hormones

Hormones are chemicals produced by endocrine glands that regulate the function of different organs and systems in our body. In particular, hormones play an important role in regulating the immune system. For example, cortisol is a hormone released by the adrenal gland during times of stress that helps to suppress inflammation. The thyroid hormones help to modulate the sensitivity of certain cells to infection and regulate the production of cytokines. In addition, sex hormones such as testosterone and estrogen play a role in modulating the immune response, including influencing the types of antibodies produced. Thus, hormones are essential for maintaining a healthy balance between inflammation and immunity in our body.

Although hormones are important for the regulation of the immune system, they can also lead to dysregulation. For instance, high levels of cortisol can suppress the immune response too much and make it difficult for our body to fight off infections. Additionally, fluctuations in sex hormone levels can also result in an increased risk of autoimmune diseases such as lupus or rheumatoid arthritis. Therefore, it is important to ensure that our hormones remain balanced in order to maintain a healthy immune system.

The endocrine system also plays an important role in aging, which can affect the function of the immune system. As we age, there are changes in hormone production and levels that can impair the ability of our body to protect itself from infection and disease. For example, older adults tend to produce less cortisol and other hormones that help regulate the immune system. Therefore, maintaining hormonal balance is essential for promoting healthy aging and a strong immune system.

What Are The Types Of Hormones?

Hormones are classified into several categories based on their structure and function. The three main classes of hormones are steroid, peptide, and amine hormones.

Steroid Hormones

Steroid hormones are lipid-soluble molecules that include glucocorticoids, mineralocorticoids, and sex hormones. Glucocorticoids are secreted by the adrenal cortex and help to regulate metabolism and fight stress. Mineralocorticoids, such as aldosterone, are produced in the adrenal gland and help to regulate electrolyte balance. Sex hormones, such as testosterone and estrogen, are produced in the testes and ovaries, respectively, and help to regulate sexual development and reproductive function.

Peptide Hormones

Peptide hormones are short chains of amino acids that are secreted by glands such as the pituitary gland or pancreas. Examples include growth hormone (GH), insulin, and cholecystokinin (CCK). GH is involved in growth and development. Insulin helps to regulate blood sugar levels by promoting the transport of glucose into cells. CCK stimulates the release of digestive enzymes from the pancreas.

Amine Hormones

Amine hormones are derived from amino acids and include epinephrine (adrenaline), norepinephrine, and thyroxine. Epinephrine is secreted by the adrenal glands in response to stress, while norepinephrine helps to regulate metabolism and alertness. Thyroxine is produced in the thyroid gland and helps to regulate metabolic rate.

Hormones play a crucial role in regulating the immune system. In order to ensure a healthy and balanced immune response, it is important to maintain proper levels of hormones. In addition, understanding how hormones affect the different components of the immune system can help us better understand and treat immunological disorders.

Chemical Mechanisms Of Hormones

Hormones play a crucial role in the regulation of the immune system by means of chemical signaling. Hormones are secreted either directly into the blood or bound to carrier proteins and then released into circulation when needed. When hormones reach their target cells, they bind to specific receptors located on the outer membrane of the cells. This binding triggers a cascade of chemical reactions inside the cell, resulting in a response. For example, when cortisol binds to its receptor, it triggers the release of an enzyme that helps to suppress inflammation. Similarly, testosterone and estrogen bind to their respective receptors and trigger different responses depending on the type of cell they are targeting.

In addition to direct chemical signaling through hormones, the immune system is also regulated by indirect mechanisms. For instance, hormones can affect the production of cytokines, which play a key role in modulating the immune response. Cytokines are released by cells in response to certain stimuli and help to regulate inflammation and immunity. Thus, hormones act as an important control mechanism for the immune system by influencing the production of cytokines.

Finally, hormone production can also be regulated by the functioning of other hormones. For instance, cortisol levels are affected by adrenaline and thyroxine, which help to regulate how much cortisol is released. Thus, hormones interact with each other in complex ways that affect the overall balance of the immune system.

Physical Mechanisms Of Hormones

In addition to chemical signaling, hormones also have physical effects on the body that help regulate the immune system. For instance, cortisol can inhibit inflammation by reducing blood flow to inflamed tissues. Testosterone and estrogen can increase or decrease local concentrations of certain immune cells based on their hormone levels. Finally, growth hormone has been found to influence lymphocyte production and maturation.

B Lymphocytes

B Lymphocytes are a type of white blood cell in the immune system that defend against bacteria and viruses. They produce proteins known as antibodies, which attach to foreign invaders and mark them for destruction by other cells.

When B Cells encounter an antigen, they form clones and undergo a process of selection and maturation. This allows them to develop receptors that are specific to particular antigens and leads to the development of memory B Cells. Memory cells help the body recognize when an antigen is encountered again, resulting in a more rapid response time.

B Lymphocytes also play an important role in humoral immunity by helping proteins called complements bind to invaders, leading to their destruction. They also help activate T cells, a type of white blood cell that plays a key role in the adaptive immune response.

In addition, B Lymphocytes are responsible for producing cytokines, small proteins that regulate communication between cells and help direct the immune response. They also produce large amounts of antibodies which can be used to neutralize toxins and viruses before they cause damage. Lastly, B Cells are capable of presenting antigens to T Cells, which then initiate an antigen-specific response.

T Cells

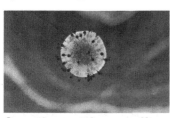

T cells are an important part of the immune system as they have a diverse range of functions. These cells can identify and eliminate virus infected or cancerous cells, control other elements of the immune response, and even play roles in allergic reactions.

T cells have receptors that bind to specific antigens on foreign objects, such as viruses or bacteria. This binding initiates a response by the T cells that can either directly kill the intruder or stimulate other components of the immune system to do so.

Additionally, T cells can produce cytokines, which are molecules that help coordinate and modulate the overall immune response.

T cells can be divided into several categories based on their function: helper T cells, killer T cells, and regulatory T cells. Helper T cells are important for activating other components of the immune system, including B cells which produce antibodies to fight bacteria or viruses. Killer T cells directly kill infected or cancerous cells through a process known as apoptosis. Finally, Regulatory T Cells help to balance the immune response by suppressing over-active immune responses which can cause autoimmunity.

The diverse range of functions of T cells makes them an important component for maintaining a healthy immune system and protecting us from foreign invaders. Without these cells, our body would be unable to effectively fight off disease-causing pathogens, which could lead to serious illness or death.

Phagocytes And Their Relatives

Phagocytes and their relatives are one of the most important components of the immune system. Phagocytes engulf and digest invading pathogens, activating other cells in the process. These cells include macrophages, dendritic cells, neutrophils, and eosinophils. Macrophages are found throughout the body and act as scavengers by ingesting and destroying cellular debris. Dendritic cells are specialized to detect foreign particles and activate other components of the immune system. Neutrophils and eosinophils work together to attack invading pathogens directly by releasing toxic molecules.

In addition, phagocytes can also release cytokines that help regulate the immune response. Cytokines are proteins that help regulate various aspects of the immune system, including inflammation and cell-to-cell communication. Cytokines support the growth and development of many cells within the immune system, including B lymphocytes and T lymphocytes. These cells are responsible for producing antibodies that can recognize foreign invaders and direct other components of the immune system to attack them.

As a result, the complex combination of phagocytes and their relatives plays an essential role in maintaining a healthy immune system. By engulfing, destroying, and signaling to other components of the immune system, these cells are able to protect our bodies from invading pathogens. Without them, the body would be vulnerable to attack from foreign invaders.

Phagocytes and their relatives can also play a role in autoimmunity, when the immune system begins to attack the body's own tissues. In these cases, certain components of the immune system become overactive and begin attacking healthy cells or organs. By understanding how phagocytes work and recognizing signs of an overactive immune response, it is possible to prevent and treat autoimmune diseases such as lupus or rheumatoid arthritis.

Overall, phagocytes and their relatives are a fundamental component of the immune system, providing our bodies with essential protection from harm. By understanding how they work and recognizing signs of an overactive response, it is possible to maintain a healthy immune system and prevent autoimmune diseases.

Self And Nonself

The human immune system is designed to identify and attack foreign substances, such as viruses and bacteria, that it considers to be harmful. To do this, the immune system must be able to distinguish between the body's own cells and molecules (known as "self") and those of an invading organism (known as "nonself").

What Is The Meaning Of Self And Nonself?

Self and nonself are terms used to describe the distinction made by the human immune system between its own cells and molecules (known as "self") and those of an invading organism (known as "nonself"). This distinction is crucial for our bodies to be able to fight off pathogens. The body produces antibodies which help it recognize these foreign substances and either destroy them or alert the body's immune system. Without this distinction, our bodies would not be able to effectively fight off invading pathogens.

The ability of the immune system to distinguish between self and nonself is a product of evolution and has allowed us to survive despite exposure to many different viruses and bacteria over time. It is one of the most important aspects of our immune system and one that we rely upon to keep us healthy.

In order for the self vs. nonself distinction to be effective, it must remain highly specific. Our bodies are constantly exposed to foreign substances which can potentially harm us, and the immune system must be able to identify these quickly and efficiently in order to protect us from infection. In the case of autoimmune diseases, however, this process fails and our bodies end up attacking our own cells. Autoimmune diseases can be very serious and often require lifelong treatment in order to keep them under control.

The self vs. nonself distinction is a complex system which has developed over millions of years in order for us to survive despite exposure to potentially harmful foreign substances. It is a crucial part of our immune system and one that we rely on to keep us healthy. Without it, many diseases would be much more common and our bodies would not be able to fight off infection as effectively.

Innate Immunity

Innate immunity is the first line of defense a body has to fight off infections and diseases. It is an evolutionarily ancient system that works by recognizing any foreign particles, such as viruses or bacteria, that enter the body. This allows the body to quickly respond and create an immune response before these pathogens have a chance to spread throughout the body or cause infection.

Innate immunity is made up of physical barriers, like the skin and mucous membranes, as well as chemical signals from certain cells that can help alert the body to an infection. When a pathogen enters the body, special immune cells present in the bloodstream recognize it and release cytokines. These molecules then travel through the bloodstream and activate other parts of the immune response, such as the production of antibodies.

The innate immune system is also involved in helping to regulate inflammation. This process is important for keeping infections from spreading too far and preventing long-term damage to tissues. The body's upregulation of inflammatory markers helps to alert other components of the immune system to help fight off any potential threats. Innate immunity also plays an essential role in helping the body to recognize and distinguish between whether something is a friend or foe, allowing it to respond appropriately.

Innate immunity is a powerful first line of defense that helps protect us from many different pathogens. It's important to remember, however, that while innate immunity can help fight off infection, it alone cannot completely rid the body of all pathogens. That's why having a strong adaptive immune system is essential for maintaining good health.

Chemical Mechanisms Of Innate Immunity

Chemical mechanisms of Innate Immunity involve the release of special molecules called cytokines. These molecules are produced by certain immune cells and travel throughout the body to activate other parts of the immune system, such as producing antibodies or activating other cells involved in fighting off infection.

In addition to cytokines, there are also a number of other chemical agents involved in Innate Immunity. These include antibodies, complement proteins, and antimicrobial peptides. Antibodies are important for recognizing and targeting specific foreign particles, while complement proteins help to activate other parts of the immune system that can fight off infection. Antimicrobial peptides also help to destroy any pathogens that manage to make it past the physical barriers of the body.

Physical Mechanisms Of Innate Immunity

Physical mechanisms of Innate Immunity involve the use of physical barriers such as the skin and mucous membranes. These barriers help to protect the body from any foreign particles that may enter, preventing them from entering into deeper tissues or organs. If these pathogens do manage to make it through these physical barriers, cells called phagocytes can surround and engulf them, helping to protect the body from further infection.

In addition, special cells called macrophages are also involved in helping to regulate inflammation. These cells help to alert other parts of the immune system when a pathogen enters the body and can also release cytokines that activate other parts of the immune response. Ultimately, these physical barriers combined with cell-mediated responses work together to help protect the body from infection.

The innate immune system is a powerful first line of defense that helps to protect us from many different pathogens. It involves both physical and chemical mechanisms that work together to keep us safe from infection. While it can't completely rid the body of all pathogens, it does play an essential role in keeping our bodies healthy and functioning properly.

In addition to protecting us from infection, the

innate immune system also plays an important role in helping the body distinguish between what is friend or foe. This helps ensure that the body only reacts to foreign particles and doesn't mistakenly attack its own cells or tissues. Innate immunity is essential for maintaining good health and without it, we would be much more vulnerable to infections and diseases.

Adaptive Immunity

Adaptive immunity is the branch of the immune system that allows for vaccination and long-term memory. It's what makes our bodies able to recognize and fight against pathogens it has seen before.

It works by identifying antigens on a pathogen, which are molecules that can be recognized by specialized cells called lymphocytes. These lymphocytes produce antibodies that attach to the antigens and cause their destruction. The lymphocytes also remember antigens from previous encounters, which allows us to build immunity over time.

Vaccines work by using a weakened or dead version of the pathogen that triggers an immune response without causing illness. This produces memory cells that are able to recognize and fight off the virus if we're ever exposed to it again.

Adaptive immunity is essential for protecting us against dangerous pathogens and allowing us to develop immunity over time. It's one of the most powerful tools in our fight against disease.

Chemical Mechanisms Of Adaptive Immunity

In addition to generating specific antibodies, adaptive immunity also uses a number of chemical mechanisms to fight off pathogens. One of the most important is complement activation, which is a cascade of reactions that leads to the destruction of antigens by forming holes in their cell membranes. This enables them to be attacked by phagocytes, which are specialized immune cells that eat and destroy invading pathogens.

Another mechanism is cytokine production, which are chemicals that help to coordinate the immune response by attracting other cells and molecules to the site of infection. This helps to create a stronger defense against invaders and can reduce the severity and duration of an illness.

Finally, adaptive immunity also uses toll-like receptor signalling, where specialized receptors on cells recognize molecules of pathogens and alert the immune system to their presence. This helps to initiate an even stronger, more rapid response that can help to protect us from serious illness.

Physical Mechanisms Of Adaptive Immunity

Adaptive immunity also utilizes physical mechanisms to attack pathogens. It does this through a process called phagocytosis, where specialized immune cells known as phagocytes engulf and digest invading pathogens. The phagocytes then release chemicals that can help to further destroy the pathogen or alert other immune cells to its presence.

Another physical mechanism is lymphocyte activation, which is when specialized lymphocytes recognize antigens on a pathogen and activate other immune cells to fight them off. This helps to create a stronger defense against invaders that can help us to better protect ourselves against illness.

All of these physical and chemical mechanisms work together to create an effective adaptive immunity system that can help us stay healthy in the face of pathogens.

What Are Some Ways Of Helping The Body Distinguish Between Self And Nonself?

One way of helping the body to distinguish between self and nonself is through vaccination. Vaccines are essentially harmless versions of a pathogen which help the body to learn how to fight off that particular disease in the future. By exposing our bodies to these foreign substances, their immune systems can begin to recognize them as nonself and create antibodies which will then attack them if they ever enter the body again. This helps protect us from potentially deadly illnesses.

Immunotherapy is another way of helping the

body distinguish between self and non-self. In this type of treatment, doctors use substances such as antibodies or other molecules to encourage the body's immune system to recognize certain foreign substances as nonself and destroy them. This can be used for both acute and chronic conditions, such as cancer or autoimmune diseases.

Finally, another way of helping the body distinguish between self and nonself is by maintaining a healthy lifestyle. Eating a balanced diet, getting regular exercise, and keeping stress levels low can all help to keep our immune systems functioning properly. This will enable them to more effectively recognize foreign substances as nonself and fight off any invading pathogens.

CHAPTER 3: FUNCTIONS OF THE IMMUNE SYSTEM

1. Pathogen recognition and response

Pathogen recognition and response is a major function of the immune system. In order to protect the body from harmful pathogens, such as bacteria and viruses, it has developed an array of tools that enable it to recognize and destroy them. Pathogens can be recognized by the innate immune system using pattern recognition receptors (PRRs) or by antibodies produced by the adaptive immune system. Upon recognition, both systems trigger an inflammatory response to help eliminate the pathogen and restore homeostasis. In addition, certain components of the immune system facilitate the clearance of dead cells or debris that can result from a pathogenic infection. As such, it is clear that maintaining a healthy immune system is essential for avoiding disease and staying healthy.

2. Eliminating Abnormal Or Damaged Cells

The immune system also helps to protect the body from itself by recognizing and destroying abnormal or damaged cells, such as cancerous cells. This process is known as immunosurveillance, and it involves the recognition of aberrant molecules on cell surfaces that are not typically found in healthy cells. When these molecules are identified, appropriate defense mechanisms can be triggered to destroy the affected cells.

The immune system also plays an important role in controlling inflammation in the body. Inflammation helps the body to respond and heal from injury, but too much of it can damage healthy tissue. To protect against this, the immune system releases cytokines that help to regulate the inflammatory response while allowing healing to occur.

Finally, the immune system plays an important role in maintaining overall health and wellness by modulating a healthy stress response. Stress hormones, such as cortisol, are released during times of stress and can have a negative impact on the body if left unchecked. The immune system helps to regulate these hormones, allowing for a balanced response that doesn't overwhelm the body.

By recognizing, responding to, and eliminating foreign substances, abnormal cells, and excess inflammation in the body, the immune system is a crucial component of our overall health and well-being. Taking care of your immune system is key to keeping your body healthy.

3. Protection From Infection

The immune system is the body's first line of

defence against infection. It consists of several components that work together to protect us from harm. The immune system can recognize and respond to foreign substances, such as bacteria or viruses, and remove them before they can cause disease.

The primary way in which the body defends itself against infection is by producing antibodies. Antibodies are proteins produced by the body in response to a foreign substance and help to identify and destroy it. The body also produces other types of cells, such as T-cells and B-cells, which play an important role in fighting infection.

In addition, the immune system uses white blood cells to help fight infections. White blood cells can recognize and destroy bacteria or viruses that enter the body, and they also help to activate other parts of the immune system.

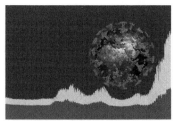 The immune system is a complex network of organs and cells, all working together to protect us from infection. By understanding how it functions, we can better understand how to keep our bodies healthy and prevent illness. Vaccines are an important way to do this as they help to educate and train the immune system, so it can recognize and fight off infection before it takes hold.

Immune Memory

Immune memory is the ability of the immune system to remember and quickly recognize a specific pathogen that it has previously encountered. It helps our body fight the same infection more effectively in future by preparing us ahead of time. This process involves white blood cells called B-cells and T-cells which are responsible for recognizing pathogens, forming an immunological memory and responding to them more quickly and efficiently. By generating immunological memory, the body can generate an effective response to a pathogen with fewer resources than if it had never encountered the pathogen before. This is why vaccines are so effective — they introduce antigens into our bodies in order to create immunity without exposing us to the disease itself.

Immune memory helps protect us from both new and old infections, by allowing our bodies to quickly recognize and respond to them. As we age, our immune system may no longer be able to fight off new infections as effectively as it did when we were younger. This is why older people are more susceptible to certain diseases and illnesses. However, having an immunological memory can help protect us even in later life by allowing us to mount an effective response against a certain pathogen with fewer resources.

Immune memory is also important for protecting us from chronic infections such as HIV or the herpes virus, which can persist in our bodies for many years. By having immunological memory, the body can recognize and respond more quickly to these pathogens even after long periods of latency. This is why treatments such as antiretrovirals are so important for treating these types of infections — they help the body to recognize and fight off the virus more efficiently.

Immune memory is one of the most important functions of our immune system, as it helps protect us from both new and old pathogens by allowing us to respond to them quickly and effectively. Vaccines are a great way to form immunological memory and should be taken regularly in order to maintain optimal health. For those suffering from chronic infections, antiretrovirals may be necessary in order to help the body recognize and fight off the virus more efficiently. Additionally, it is important to ensure that our bodies have adequate nutrition and rest in order to keep our immune system functioning optimally. Doing so will help ensure that our immune system can form immunological memory and maintain a strong defense against pathogens of all types.

What Is The Role Of B-Cells And T-Cells In Creating Immunological Memory?

The primary role of B-cells and T-cells in the formation of immunological memory is to recognize pathogens and then activate the immune system to create an effective response. B-cells produce antibodies which are used to bind to antigens on the surface of pathogens, helping the body to recognize them as foreign entities. T-cells, meanwhile, can recognize antigens that have been processed by other cells in the body and help activate other parts of the immune system such as cytokines.

When the immune system encounters a pathogen, B-cells and T-cells become activated and produce proteins called memory cells, which are specific to that particular pathogen. These memory cells help the body to remember and recognize the pathogen in future so that it can respond more quickly and effectively if it is encountered again. This process is essential for creating immunological memory, as it allows the body to recognize and respond to a pathogen more quickly and efficiently than if it had never encountered the pathogen before.

Overall, B-cells and T-cells play an important role in creating immunological memory by recognizing pathogens and triggering an effective immune response. This process is essential for protecting us against both new and old infections and is a key function of our immune system. Vaccines are an effective way to create immunological memory without exposing us to the disease itself. Additionally, antiretrovirals and other treatments may be necessary for creating immunity against chronic infections such as HIV or the herpes virus. Finally, it is important to ensure that our bodies have adequate nutrients and rest in order to keep our immune system functioning optimally and help it create a strong defense against pathogens of all types.

What Are The Benefits Of Having An Immunological Memory?

The main benefit of having an immunological memory is that it helps our body fight the same infection more effectively in future by preparing us ahead of time. This allows us to mount an effective response to a pathogen with fewer resources than if it had never encountered the pathogen before. This is why vaccines are so effective—they introduce antigens into our bodies in order to create immunity without exposing us to the disease itself. Additionally, having immunological memory helps protect us from chronic infections which can persist in our bodies for many years, as the body can recognize and respond more quickly to these pathogens even after long periods of latency.

Immune memory is also important for protecting us from new infections, as our bodies may no longer be able to fight off certain infections as effectively as it did when we were younger. By having immunological memory, our body can mount an effective response against a certain pathogen more quickly and efficiently. Finally, having a strong immunological memory can help us maintain optimal health and protect us from many types of diseases and illnesses.

Metabolic Functions

Metabolic functions refer to the actions that immune cells perform in order to maintain homeostasis within the body. These include producing cytokines and other proteins that regulate inflammation, as well as releasing enzymes which break down foreign molecules. They also help with cell divisions and DNA repair, ensuring that healthy cells remain viable. Additionally, metabolic functions are responsible for activating or suppressing certain pathways which influence cell development and growth. This ensures that the immune system can respond quickly and effectively to invading pathogens. Ultimately, metabolic functions help keep our bodies healthy and functioning properly.

In addition to homeostatic activities, metabolic functions also play an important role in the body's response against particular infections or foreign substances. When certain molecules are identified as being harmful or potentially dangerous, the immune system will activate a specific metabolic pathway to neutralize and detoxify the threat. This helps protect us from potential illness or disease.

Metabolic functions are essential for maintaining a healthy balance within our bodies. Without them, we would be vulnerable to various illnesses and infections due to an inability to effectively fight off foreign invaders. It is therefore important that we keep our metabolic functions functioning properly in order to stay healthy.

Homeostasis

Homeostasis is the ability of an organism to regulate its internal environment in order to maintain a state of equilibrium on different levels. It is an essential function of the immune system, which helps keep the body healthy by maintaining balance and defending against harmful pathogens. The immune system works in concert with other bodily systems to monitor changes in the internal environment and respond accordingly to maintain homeostasis. It is made up of several components, including the lymphatic system, which consists of white blood cells and antibodies that attack foreign invaders; the digestive tract, which absorbs nutrients from food to fuel the body; and the endocrine system, which produces hormones that help regulate bodily functions. These components work together to protect against disease-causing organisms and keep the body healthy.

In order for homeostasis to occur, the immune system must be able to recognize and identify foreign substances, such as bacteria or viruses, that can cause harm. It does this through a process known as antigen recognition, where cells bind to antigens on the surface of the invading organism and then activate other components of the immune system to fight the infection or disease.

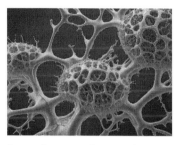 The immune system also plays an important role in allergies and autoimmune diseases, when it mistakenly identifies a harmless substance as a foreign invader and produces antibodies to attack it. This can lead to inflammation, rashes, breathing problems, and other symptoms. The immune response can be affected by things like stress levels and nutrition, so it is important to take care of your body and mind to ensure that the immune system is functioning optimally.

Finally, the immune system contributes to overall health by producing cytokines, proteins that act as chemical messengers between cells and help regulate many bodily processes such as inflammation. These cytokines can help promote healing and protect against disease-causing organisms. By keeping the body in a balanced state, homeostasis is an important part of maintaining good health.

Tolerance

Tolerance is the ability of the immune system to distinguish between self and nonself molecules. It helps the body distinguish between healthy, normal cells and foreign invaders like viruses or bacteria. When the body encounters something it recognizes as foreign, it launches an immune response to get rid of it. Tolerance allows these responses to be very specific, meaning they can target only certain cells or molecules. This helps the body avoid attacking its own healthy, normal cells and maintain a balanced immune system.

The immune system needs to remain tolerant in order to stay healthy. When the body encounters something it doesn't recognize as foreign, it can cause an autoimmune response, where the immune system mistakenly attacks its own healthy cells. This can lead to a wide range of health issues, including allergies, asthma, and autoimmune diseases.

In order to maintain tolerance, the body needs to be regularly exposed to foreign substances in order to remain accustomed to them. This is why vaccines are important – they introduce small amounts of a virus or bacteria into the body so that it can recognize it as friendly and strengthen its immune response to it should the body ever encounter a larger amount. Vaccines are an important part of keeping the immune system tolerant and healthy.

Immunological Surveillance

Immunological surveillance is the process by which a person's body monitors for foreign invaders like viruses, bacteria, and other pathogens. It involves various molecules and cells of the immune system that identify potentially dangerous agents in the body and then launch an appropriate response to neutralize or eliminate them before they cause harm. This includes both innate (non-specific) mechanisms such as physical barriers like skin and mucus, as well as specific (adaptive) processes such as the production of antibodies that recognize and bind to pathogens. Immunological surveillance is essential for maintaining a healthy immune system and preventing infection or disease. It can also play an important role in detecting cancerous cells before they spread. Overall, immunological surveillance helps keep us safe from harm and provides a powerful layer of protection from disease.

Immunological surveillance is closely linked with immunization, which is the process of deliberately introducing an antigen to the body in order to stimulate an immune response and provide immunity against a particular pathogen. By introducing small amounts of an antigen (e.g., a vaccine), the body can be taught how to recognize it and launch an appropriate response in the event of a future infection. This process helps protect us from diseases like measles, influenza, hepatitis, and other life-threatening illnesses.

Immunological surveillance is also important for diagnosing autoimmune diseases such as rheumatoid arthritis or type 1 diabetes. In these cases, the immune system mistakenly attacks healthy tissues instead of foreign invaders, leading to inflammation and other immune-related symptoms. By monitoring the body for signs of aberrant immunological activity, doctors can more accurately diagnose these conditions and begin treatment as soon as possible.

Immunoprotection

Immunoprotection is the process of protecting an organism from disease by stimulating or improving its immunological response. This can be done through a variety of means, such as vaccination, which prepares the body for potential exposure to disease; administration of antibodies that can target and neutralize disease-causing agents; or genetic engineering to enhance the effectiveness of an individual's immune system. In general, immunoprotection is a key factor in maintaining health and preventing infection, as it helps the body to recognize foreign substances that may be harmful and mount an appropriate defense. Immunoprotection is also important for improving the effectiveness of therapies such as chemotherapy, which can weaken the immune system. Understanding how immunoprotection works can provide insight into the development and spread of infectious diseases, as well as help to develop treatments for such diseases.

In general, immunoprotection is a complex physiological process that can be divided into two main categories: innate and adaptive immunity. Innate immunity refers to a body's natural ability to recognize foreign substances quickly and deploy appropriate defense mechanisms against them. Adaptive immunity is more specific, as it involves the body's production of specific antibodies to target particular pathogens. Both forms of immunoprotection can be enhanced through vaccination, and this is one of the most common methods used to protect individuals from infectious diseases.

Immunoprotection can also be improved through genetic engineering techniques, in which genes that encode for certain proteins or molecules that allow the body to recognize antigens and produce the antibodies needed to fight them are inserted into an individual's genome. This approach has been used in the development of treatments for various types of cancer, as well as infectious diseases such as HIV/AIDS.

CHAPTER 4: FACTORS AFFECTING IMMUNE SYSTEM HEALTH

Factors affecting immune system health

Your immune system is an essential part of your body, and it's important to understand what can affect your health. Many factors can have a negative impact on our immune systems, some of which include:

How Does Nutrition Affect Immune Response?

Nutrition plays an important role in maintaining a healthy immune system, as certain vitamins and minerals can support its function. Eating a balanced diet that includes a variety of fruits, vegetables, whole grains, and proteins can help ensure that the body is getting all the nutrients it needs to maintain homeostasis and fight off invading organisms.

Certain foods are particularly beneficial for immune health; they include:

- Fruits and vegetables are high in antioxidants: These help reduce inflammation and boost immunity. Examples include blueberries, oranges, spinach, and broccoli.
- Omega-3 fatty acids: These are found in fish such as salmon and sardines and have anti-inflammatory effects.

- Probiotics: These are live bacteria that can help support the gut microbiome, which is important for a healthy immune system. They can be found in fermented foods like yoghurt and kimchi.
- Vitamin C: This vitamin is important for many immune system functions, and can be found in citrus fruits, bell peppers, broccoli, and Brussels sprouts.
- Zinc: This mineral plays a role in wound healing and fighting infection, and is found in foods such as oysters, nuts, beans, and seeds.

In addition to consuming a healthy diet, staying hydrated is important for immune health as it helps the body flush out toxins. Getting sufficient exercise and sleep also helps keep the immune system functioning optimally.

By following these simple guidelines, you can help ensure that your body has the resources it needs to maintain homeostasis and protect against disease-causing organisms. Taking care of your body is an essential part of staying healthy and keeping the immune system working properly.

Stress

Stress has long been known to have a negative effect on overall health, but it also affects our immune system. Studies have shown that stress can weaken the body's natural defenses against viruses, bacteria, and other pathogens. It can also slow down the body's response to infection.

The effects of chronic stress are especially damaging to the immune system. Chronic stress can disrupt the normal activity of our cells, leading to a weakened immune response and greater susceptibility to infections. It's important to find ways to reduce your levels of stress in order to maintain good health and protect against illness. Exercise, meditation, yoga, journaling and other relaxation techniques can all help manage stress levels and support a healthy immune system.

Additionally, it's a good idea to get sufficient sleep. Sleep is an important part of the body's recovery process, as it helps repair the immune system and supports energy levels. Aiming for 8 hours per night can help keep your immune system in good working order by giving your body the chance to restore itself.

How Does Lack Of Sleep Affect The Immune System?

It's well established that lack of sleep can have a negative impact on your immune system. When you don't get adequate rest, it takes a toll on your body and makes it more vulnerable to infection and disease. A few hours here or there may not seem like much, but consistently depriving yourself of quality sleep will leave you more susceptible to catching a cold or other illnesses.

Sleep deprivation weakens your immune system in a few different ways: it reduces the production of antibodies and cytokines, which are molecules that help fight infection; it also decreases the number of T-cells, which are important for fighting off viruses and bacteria. Additionally, lack of sleep increases levels of stress hormones like cortisol, which can suppress your immune system's response to germs.

There are several lifestyle changes you can make to get more quality sleep and improve your immune system health: avoid caffeine late in the day, create a relaxing nighttime routine, keep consistent bedtimes and wake times (even on the weekends!), limit screen time before bed, and exercise regularly. If you're having trouble falling asleep or staying asleep, your doctor may be able to help.

Getting enough restful sleep is one of the best ways to keep your immune system functioning optimally and fend off illnesses.

How Does Smoking Or Drinking Alcohol Affect The Immune System?

Smoking and drinking alcohol both have a negative effect on the immune system. Smoking compromises its ability to defend against airborne pathogens, while alcohol destroys healthy cells and impairs the body's ability to respond to foreign invaders.

The most direct way that smoking affects the immune system is by decreasing the body's natural defenses against disease-causing bacteria and viruses. Cigarette smoke contains toxic compounds such as tar, carbon monoxide and polycyclic aromatic hydrocarbons, which can damage the respiratory system by making it more vulnerable to infection. In addition, smoking decreases the effectiveness of macrophages, a type of white blood cell that is essential for fighting off invading bacteria and viruses.

Alcohol affects the immune system in a different way. It suppresses the production of proteins and hormones that are essential for fighting off infection and decreases the effectiveness of antibodies. In addition, it causes inflammation which can impair the body's natural healing processes. Heavy drinking is especially damaging to the immune system as it increases the risk of developing illnesses such as pneumonia, tuberculosis, or sepsis.

To ensure optimal immune system health, it is important to avoid smoking and limit the consumption of alcohol. Eating a balanced diet that includes foods high in vitamins, minerals, and antioxidants can also help promote healthy immunity. Regular physical activity has been found to reduce inflammation and improve overall immune system functioning. By following these guidelines, you can take steps towards improving your body's natural defenses against illness and disease.

How Do Certain Medications Affect The Immune System?

Certain medications can have a direct effect on the functioning of your immune system. Some medications, such as corticosteroids and chemotherapy drugs, are known to suppress the activity of the immune system. This means that people taking these medications may be more prone to illnesses and infections. Other medication classes, such as antibiotics and antifungals, are designed to target specific organisms that may cause infections. While these medications can help fight off infection, they also have the potential to weaken your immune system by killing beneficial bacteria in your body. It is important to discuss the potential side effects of any medications with your doctor before taking them. Taking supplements to support and maintain a healthy immune system can also help counter the effects of certain medications on your immune system.

Additionally, certain lifestyle choices can also have an effect on the functioning of your immune system. Poor dietary habits, sedentary lifestyles, and smoking can lower the efficacy of your immune system's defenses. Therefore, it is important to lead a healthy lifestyle in order to promote good immune health. Eating a balanced diet that includes fresh fruits and vegetables, lean proteins, and healthy fats is essential for supporting your immune system. Regular exercise can also help keep your immune system in check, as it helps to reduce stress and improves overall health. Finally, staying away from smoking can both improve your health and boost the effectiveness of your immune system. All of these factors combine to help maintain a strong and healthy immune system that is capable of fighting off disease and infection.

It is important to note that the effectiveness of your immune system can also be affected by age and genetics. People with a weakened immune system, such as those living with HIV/AIDS or undergoing chemotherapy, may need to take added precautions to protect their health. Additionally, older adults often have weaker immune systems than younger people, so they may need to take additional steps to ensure their health. Ultimately, it is important to be mindful of your overall health and lifestyle habits in order to maintain a healthy immune system.

How Do Toxins And Pollutants Affect The Immune System?

The presence of toxins and pollutants in the environment can have an adverse effect on our immune system. Chemicals, such as heavy metals like lead and mercury, volatile organic compounds (VOCs), and polychlorinated biphenyls (PCBs) can interfere with the body's ability to fight off disease-causing pathogens. In addition, exposure to these chemicals can cause inflammation and oxidative stress, which can further weaken the immune system. Additionally, some of these toxins may impact the development of our bodies' lymphocytes, which are a key component in fighting infections.

To reduce exposure to toxins and pollutants, make sure that your environment is as clean as possible by regularly vacuuming or dusting and using air filters. Additionally, look for products that are free of toxins and pollutants, such as organic foods and household items. Finally, be sure to get regular medical checkups in order to screen for any health issues related to exposure to toxins and pollutants. By taking these simple steps, you can help protect your immune system from the negative effects of environmental toxins and pollutants.

By making sure that we focus on healthy habits such as eating a balanced diet, getting enough sleep and exercise, managing stress levels and avoiding smoking and drinking alcohol, we can help to keep our immune systems strong. By staying mindful of these factors, we can ensure that our bodies are able to protect us from illness and disease.

Immunodeficiency Disorders

Immunodeficiency disorders are conditions in

which the immune system is impaired or non-functioning. These disorders can be caused by genetic defects, environmental factors (such as exposure to certain toxins), and acquired infections that suppress the proper functioning of the immune system. Common symptoms of immunodeficiencies include frequent bacterial and fungal infections, recurrent viral illnesses, and susceptibility to certain types of cancer.

Immunodeficiencies can be divided into two broad categories: primary and secondary immunodeficiencies. Primary immunodeficiencies are inherited conditions that disrupt the development, structure, or function of the immune system. Examples include severe combined immunodeficiency (SCID) and Wiskott–Aldrich Syndrome (WAS). Secondary immunodeficiencies are acquired conditions that occur after birth and can be caused by certain medications, radiation therapy, or infection with a virus such as HIV/AIDS.

Challenges Faced By The Immune System

Drug Resistance In Pathogens

The immune system faces a daunting challenge in the form of drug resistance in pathogens. Drug resistance is when bacteria, viruses, and other pathogenic organisms become resistant to medication meant to fight them. This can occur naturally or through the overuse of antibiotics, which encourages the selection of antibiotic-resistant strains of these organisms.

Drug resistance has increased significantly over the last few decades, leading to a rise in multi-drug-resistant infections. This is a serious public health issue as more and more common illnesses become harder to treat with traditional medications.

In order to combat drug resistance, scientists and healthcare professionals must take steps to limit the use of antibiotics and other medications whenever possible. Vaccines can be used to prevent diseases from occurring in the first place, and improved methods of infection control can help to limit the spread of drug-resistant bacteria.

The immune system is also being aided by advances in technology. As genetic sequencing has become more sophisticated, scientists are better able to identify microbes responsible for infections and treat them with precision medications tailored to their particular strain. This helps reduce the risk of antibiotic resistance as well as ensuring that patients receive the most effective treatment possible.

It is clear that the immune system has its work cut out for it when it comes to drug resistance, but with the right strategies and advances in technology, we can help it stay a step ahead of this formidable foe.

Probiotics: Aiding Immunity

Probiotics are being used increasingly to promote immune health. Probiotics are live microorganisms that, when consumed in adequate amounts, can have a positive effect on the gut microbiota. This helps to strengthen the body's natural defenses against infectious agents and other sources of disease.

Probiotics come in various forms, including capsules or powders that can be added to food or drinks, and fermented products such as yoghurt or kefir. Studies have shown that probiotics can help to reduce the incidence of respiratory infections, improve digestive health, and even reduce inflammation associated with chronic conditions like asthma.

Probiotics are a promising supplement for those looking to bolster their immune system. They may not be able to completely replace traditional medications, but they can provide an additional layer of protection against infectious agents.

The immune system is a complex and powerful force, but there are still ways to help it stay strong in the face of illness. With proper nutrition, exercise, and supplementation, we can all do our part to ensure that our defenses remain up to the challenge.

CHAPTER 5: DISEASE

Disease and the Immune System

The human body's immune system is incredibly complex and powerful. It has the ability to recognize thousands of foreign substances, like viruses, bacteria, and other pathogens, and develop an appropriate response to fight them off. When a person's immune system is working correctly, it can protect against many types of disease. But when it's not functioning properly or has been compromised, it can leave a person vulnerable to serious illnesses.

It's important to understand how the immune system works and what kinds of things can affect its ability to protect us from disease. There are two main components of the immune system: innate immunity and adaptive immunity. Innate immunity consists of physical barriers like skin and mucous membranes that keep pathogens out of the body, as well as chemicals and cells that can destroy invading microorganisms. Adaptive immunity is the body's more specific response to a particular pathogen, which involves the production of antibodies that are specifically targeted against that pathogen.

Diptheria

Diptheria is a highly contagious bacterial infection caused by Corynebacterium diphtheriae. It spreads through airborne particles, contact with people infected with the germ and contact with contaminated objects. Symptoms of diptheria can range from mild to severe, including sore throat, fever, swollen lymph nodes, and a thick grey or white coating on the tonsils, back of the throat or nose. In severe cases, it can cause breathing difficulties and even death. Treatment for diptheria usually includes antibiotics and supportive care. Vaccination is the best way to prevent infection.

Diptheria And The Immune System

Diphtheria is a serious disease and can lead to severe complications if it is not properly treated. A healthy immune system is essential in fighting off the bacteria that causes diphtheria, however those with weakened or compromised immune systems are more likely to be affected. Vaccination helps protect against infection, but it is important to maintain good hygiene practices such as handwashing, avoiding contact with those who are ill and staying away from large gatherings in order to minimize your risk of infection.

How Does One Develop Immunity Against Diphtheria?

The body's immune system works to protect it from infection diphtheria and other diseases.

When a person is exposed to the diphtheria bacteria, the body produces antibodies that attach themselves to the bacteria, killing it off before it can cause harm. Vaccination helps stimulate the body's immunity by introducing an active form of the bacteria into the body so that it can create its own defenses against future infection.

It is possible to develop immunity naturally through contact with the bacteria itself, however, this can be dangerous and is not recommended. Vaccination remains the safest and most effective way of protecting yourself against diphtheria.

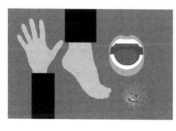

Measles

Measles is an infectious airborne virus that affects the respiratory system. It is highly contagious and can cause severe symptoms such as fever, sore throat, dry cough, runny nose, red eyes, and small white spots on the inside of the cheeks. In some cases, measles can lead to complications including pneumonia and encephalitis (brain inflammation).

Measles And The Immune System

The immune system plays a key role in resisting and combating measles. The body's natural defenses are activated when the virus enters, which triggers an inflammatory response that helps to limit its spread. The immune system produces antibodies that attack the virus, preventing it from entering cells and causing infection. Vaccinations with the measles vaccine can help stimulate the immune system to protect against future exposures to the virus. Additionally, some people who have been exposed to the measles virus may naturally develop immunity due to preexisting exposure or vaccination.

How Does One Develop Immunity Against Measles?

Immunity against measles can be developed through natural exposure to the disease, as well as through vaccination. Natural exposure occurs when the body is exposed to a weakened form of the virus, which causes it to develop antibodies that will protect against future exposures. Vaccination works in a similar way by introducing a weakened or inactive form of the virus into the body, which triggers an immune response. This process helps the body to develop immunity without experiencing the full symptoms of measles. Additionally, individuals who are vaccinated against measles may receive a booster shot periodically to ensure protection against the virus.

Mumps

Mumps is an infectious disease caused by the mumps virus. It typically begins with a few days of fever, headache, muscle aches, tiredness and loss of appetite, followed by swelling of salivary glands (parotitis). This results in the classic symptom known as "hamster face," which refers to swollen cheeks and jaw. Complications can include viral meningitis, painful swelling of the testicles or ovaries and, rarely, deafness.

Mumps And The Immune System

The mumps virus is spread through saliva and respiratory secretions, which means it is most easily spread from person-to-person contact. However, a person can also get infected by touching surfaces or objects that have been contaminated with the virus.

Once inside the body, the virus infects cells in the salivary glands and replicates itself. As the virus replicates, it triggers an immune response. The body's immune system recognizes that there is a foreign invader and responds by sending antibodies to destroy it. This process helps stop the spread of the mumps virus, but it can take up to three weeks for symptoms to appear.

In some cases, the immune system may not be able to fight off the virus. This can lead to severe cases of mumps and potential complications, such as meningitis or encephalitis. Vaccines are available that provide protection against mumps and other illnesses caused by similar viruses. By getting vaccinated, people are able to prevent these diseases from occurring and protect themselves from long-term health issues.

The best way to protect oneself against mumps is to get the vaccine. This is especially true if you live in an area where there have been recent outbreaks of mumps. If you haven't had the mumps vaccine, it's important to speak with your doctor or healthcare provider for more information and to ensure that you are up-to-date on all recommended immunizations.

How Does One Develop Immunity Against Mumps?

The immune system develops immunity to mumps by producing antibodies after being exposed to the virus. The body stores these antibodies, which allows it to recognize and respond quickly if it is exposed to the virus again. Vaccines work in a similar way by introducing a small amount of an inactive version of the virus into the body so that your immune system can recognize and respond more quickly if it is exposed to the virus in the future.

Pertussis

Pertussis, also known as whooping cough, is a highly contagious bacterial infection that affects the respiratory system. It causes severe coughing fits, which can make it difficult for people to breathe. In most cases, pertussis is treated with antibiotics or other medications. But if left untreated, it can cause serious complications, even death.

Pertussis And The Immune System

The immune system plays a crucial role in keeping us healthy and safe from many illnesses, including pertussis. When the body is exposed to an infectious agent like a bacteria or virus, the immune system responds by producing antibodies that can fight off the infection. Unfortunately, pertussis is a very contagious disease and its effects on the immune system can be quite severe.

When a person is infected with pertussis, their body produces an excessive amount of antibodies in an attempt to combat the infection. This sudden surge of antibodies weakens the immune system and makes it less effective at fighting off other illnesses. As a result, people who have been affected by pertussis are more vulnerable to other infectious agents and illnesses.

Preventing Pertussis

The best way to prevent pertussis is by getting vaccinated. Vaccines are highly effective at protecting against the disease and help to ensure that your body has the right antibodies available to fight off any potential infections. Vaccinations are particularly important for people in high-risk groups, such as infants, children under the age of five, pregnant women and people over the age of 65.

Pertussis can be especially dangerous for infants, who are too young to receive vaccinations. The best way to protect them is by making sure all people in close contact with them, such as family members and caregivers, are vaccinated. This will help to ensure that any potential infections can be contained before they reach the vulnerable infant.

In addition to vaccinating against pertussis, it is important to practice good hygiene and maintain a healthy lifestyle to help keep your immune system strong. Eating a balanced diet, getting plenty of rest, exercising regularly and avoiding contact with people who may be ill are all great ways to stay healthy.

How Does One Develop Immunity Against Pertussis?

People who have been vaccinated against pertussis will develop immunity to the disease. Vaccination stimulates the body's immune system to produce antibodies that can fight off the infection, which means that even if a person is exposed to pertussis, their body will be able to recognize and combat it before they become sick.

In some cases, people may develop immunity to pertussis even if they have not been vaccinated. This is because the body may still produce antibodies in response to exposure to the bacteria that cause pertussis, such as Bordetella pertussis or B. parapertussis, which can provide some protection against the disease.

However, it is important to note that this type of immunity is not as strong as the immunity that comes from vaccination. Therefore, it is still best to get vaccinated in order to ensure that you are fully protected against pertussis.

The body's immunity against pertussis can also decrease over time, so it is important to make sure you stay up-to-date with your vaccinations and booster shots if necessary. Doing so will help ensure that your body has the antibodies it needs to fight off any potential infections.

Polio (Paralytic)

Polio is a highly contagious viral infection that can lead to paralysis and, in some cases, even death. It is caused by the poliovirus, which mainly affects children under five years of age. When infected, the virus enters the bloodstream and travels to the central nervous system where it damages nerve cells in the brain and spinal cord. This can cause paralysis or death, depending on the severity of the infection. To prevent this, vaccines are available that help protect against the infection. Vaccines are important because they can significantly reduce the risk of polio in children and adults alike. By getting vaccinated, people can protect themselves and their communities from this potentially devastating virus.

Furthermore, it is important to know how to

recognize signs of polio infection in order to get timely medical attention. Common signs and symptoms of polio include fever, fatigue, muscle weakness, pain or stiffness in the limbs, and difficulty breathing. If you experience any of these symptoms or suspect that someone else is infected with polio, seek medical attention immediately. Early treatment can prevent serious complications from occurring.

Polio is an insidious disease that can have devastating effects. To help ensure that everyone is protected against this deadly virus, it is important to get vaccinated and know the signs and symptoms of polio infection. By taking these steps, we can all work together to help keep our communities safe and healthy.

Polio (Paralytic) And Immune System

A healthy immune system is essential for defending against diseases, such as polio. Vaccines are a key part of maintaining immunity to the poliovirus and other illnesses. When a person gets vaccinated, it causes their body to create antibodies that can recognize and fight off the virus if they are exposed to it in the future. Additionally, getting vaccinated not only provides individual protection, but also protects the entire community by reducing the risk of an outbreak.

Immunization is one of the most cost-effective ways to protect against many illnesses, and this is especially true for diseases like polio that can cause permanent disability or death. To ensure that everyone is kept safe from these infections, individuals need to get vaccinated even if they are not traveling to an area where polio is active. This will help prevent an outbreak and protect everyone living in the area.

It is also important to take other steps to promote a healthy immune system, such as eating a balanced diet, getting regular exercise, and getting plenty of rest. These practices can strengthen the body's natural immunity against infections and help keep us safe from the serious effects of polio.

How Does One Develop Immunity Against Polio (Paralytic)?

Developing immunity to the poliovirus is key in preventing polio and its serious effects. The best way to become immune to the virus is by being vaccinated. Vaccines are effective at preventing infection and provide long-term protection against the virus.

Rubella

Rubella, also known as German Measles, is an infectious disease caused by a virus. It can cause a swelling of the lymph nodes and fever, but it usually causes a mild illness with few or no symptoms in children. However, if a pregnant woman contracts Rubella during her first trimester, she faces the risk of having her unborn child suffer from severe birth defects.

How Does Rubella Affect The Immune System?

Rubella affects the immune system by attacking and damaging cells in the lymph nodes. This leads to an inflammatory response, which triggers a fever. In most cases, the body is able to fight off the infection on its own without much damage being done. However, if Rubella invades during early pregnancy, it can cause severe birth defects such as hearing loss, cleft palate, cataracts and heart defects.

How Does One Develop Immunity Against Rubella?

A person can become immune to Rubella by getting vaccinated against it. Vaccines are available in two forms: the MMR (measles-mumps-rubella) vaccine and the monovalent rubella vaccine. Both vaccines help protect against infection with the virus, but for maximum protection, both vaccines should be given before a person becomes an adult. Additionally, if a pregnant woman has not been immunized against Rubella, she should be vaccinated as soon as possible after delivery. This will help protect both mother and baby from the potential risk of infection.

Tetanus

Tetanus is a serious and often fatal bacterial disease. It is caused by the bacterium Clostridium tetani, which can be found in soil, dust, and manure. The bacteria produce toxins that cause muscle spasms, seizures, and even death if left untreated. Tetanus can be prevented with immunization (vaccination) and treatment with antibiotics.

Most cases of tetanus occur when the bacteria enters a wound or cut in the skin, such as a puncture wound or laceration caused by stepping on a nail. It can also be acquired through contaminated surgery instruments, body piercings, and tattoos. After entering the body, it can take anywhere from 3 to 21 days for the first signs and symptoms to appear.

Common symptoms of tetanus include muscle stiffness in the neck, jaw, and other parts of the body; difficulty swallowing; fever; sweating; headache; and elevated heart rate. Treatment typically consists of antibiotics, wound care, antitoxin injections, and supportive care such as oxygen therapy or respiratory support to address breathing problems.

How Does Tetanus Affect The Immune System?

Tetanus is a bacterial disease that affects the nervous system and can be fatal if left untreated. When tetanus enters the body, it produces a toxin that interferes with nerve signals between muscles and the brain. This leads to muscle spasms, seizures, difficulty breathing, and even death in severe cases. The immune system works to fight off this infection by producing antibodies to neutralize the toxins and help clear the infection.

How Does One Develop Immunity Against Tetanus?

The primary way to protect against tetanus is through immunization (vaccination). Vaccines are available in combination with other vaccines such as diphtheria and pertussis, or they can be given separately. The vaccine induces the body's own immune system to produce antibodies that will recognize and fight off any future tetanus infection. It is recommended that individuals receive booster shots every 10 years to maintain immunity.

In addition to the vaccine, proper wound care is important in preventing tetanus infection. Wounds should be cleaned immediately and thoroughly with soap and water or a disinfectant solution to help reduce the infection risk. If wounds become infected, antibiotics may be necessary to fight off any bacteria present.

Hemophilus Influenza Type B Infection

Hemophilus influenza type B (HIB) infection is a bacterial infection caused by the bacterium Haemophilus influenzae. This bacteria can cause a range of illnesses, from mild ear infections to more severe illnesses, such as meningitis and pneumonia. HiB infections are most common in infants and young children and are typically spread through contact with an infected person, such as through coughing or sneezing. The infection can be prevented through vaccination.

How Hemophilus Influenza Type B Infection Affects The Immune System?

HiB infections can have a significant effect on the immune system. When infection occurs, it can cause inflammation, which triggers the release of cytokines and other inflammatory molecules. These molecules help to fight off the bacteria but can also damage healthy tissues in the process. In addition, HiB infection can alter the normal balance of gut microbes, leading to an overgrowth of certain bacterial species. This can lead to a weakened immune system, making it more difficult for the body to fight off other infections. HiB infection also increases the risk of developing autoimmune disorders and allergies in later life.

It is important for individuals who are at risk of contracting HiB infection to receive appropriate vaccinations as this reduces the risk of severe illness and long-term complications. Vaccination can also help to prevent the spread of infection to others. If an individual does develop symptoms, it is important to seek medical attention as soon as possible in order to receive appropriate treatment and reduce the risk of long-term complications. By staying informed about HiB infection and taking preventive steps such as vaccination, individuals can protect their health and that of their loved ones.

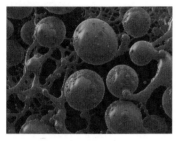

Severe Immune System Effects

In some cases, HIB infection can have serious consequences on the immune system. If not treated promptly and appropriately, it can result in sepsis, a life-threatening complication caused by an overactive immune response to an infection. It can cause organ damage and even death if left untreated. Additionally, HiB infection can lead to complications such as meningitis and bacteremia, both of which can have long-term health implications.

Since the immune system is essential for keeping us healthy, it is important to take steps to protect it from illnesses like HiB infection. Vaccination is an effective way to reduce your risk of becoming infected and prevent the spread of illness. In addition, it is important to practice good hygiene and avoid contact with anyone who may be infected. By taking these steps, individuals can help protect their own health as well as that of those around them.

How Does One Develop Immunity Against Hemophilus Influenza Type B Infection?

Immunity against HiB infection can be developed through vaccination. The HiB vaccine is typically given in three doses to create long-term immunity. It is important to ensure that all three doses are received as this helps to provide the most effective protection against HiB infection. In addition, it is also possible to develop immunity through natural exposure. This occurs when a person is exposed to the bacteria and develops an immune response. This type of immunity is typically short-term and can vary from one individual to another.

For those who may be at an increased risk of HiB infection, such as young children or individuals with weakened immune systems, vaccination is essential for protecting their health. It is also recommended for adults who have never received the vaccine or who may have been in contact with someone infected with HiB. By vaccinating and practicing good hygiene, individuals can help protect themselves from this potentially serious infection.

Hepatitis B

Hepatitis B is an infectious disease caused by the hepatitis B virus (HBV). It affects the liver and can cause both acute and chronic infections. The most serious form of HBV infection, known as fulminant hepatitis, is a rare but life-threatening condition that requires immediate medical attention. Acute hepatitis B can last for several weeks and may cause jaundice, fever, and abdominal pain. Chronic infection can last for years or even decades and may lead to cirrhosis of the liver, liver failure, or liver cancer.

HBV is spread through contact with infected blood or body fluids, such as during unprotected sexual contact or by sharing needles when injecting drugs. The virus can also be passed from mother to child during childbirth. Vaccines are available to help prevent hepatitis B. Treatment for those with chronic infection may include antiviral medications, lifestyle changes, and regular monitoring of liver function tests.

People who are at increased risk of contracting hepatitis B should be tested and vaccinated if necessary. Those who have been exposed to the virus may need a course of medication known as post-exposure prophylaxis to help prevent the virus from taking hold. Early diagnosis and treatment are important in order to reduce the risk of long-term complications. In addition, people with chronic HBV infection should be regularly monitored by their healthcare provider to ensure that their condition is being managed appropriately.

How Does Hepatitis B Affect The Immune System?

Hepatitis B can have a significant effect on the immune system. People infected with the virus are more susceptible to other infections, due to their weakened immune response. This can lead to an increased risk of developing secondary illnesses, such as bacterial and fungal infections. In addition, people with chronic hepatitis B may be at higher risk for certain cancers, including liver cancer.

In addition, people with hepatitis B may experience a range of other symptoms, including tiredness, joint pain, and loss of appetite. These can be caused by the virus's effect on the immune system and its ability to disrupt normal bodily functions. Treatment for chronic HBV infection usually involves antiviral medications that help to suppress the virus and reduce the risk of long-term complications. However, people with hepatitis B may still need to take steps to protect their overall health, such as eating a healthy diet and getting regular exercise.

How Does One Develop Immunity Against Hepatitis B?

Immunity against hepatitis B is usually achieved through vaccination. Vaccines are available to help protect people from the virus, and they can be administered either as a single dose or as a series of three doses over six months. Vaccination provides long-term protection against HBV infection and is recommended for all children aged 11–12 years old and adults at increased risk of infection.

In addition to vaccination, people can also develop immunity against hepatitis B by being naturally exposed to the virus and developing an active immune response. This is more common in regions where HBV is highly endemic, such as parts of Asia and Africa. Natural exposure may result in acute infection with a high risk of long-term complications or even death; however, it also offers lifelong protection against the virus.

Cholera

Cholera is a disease caused by the bacterium Vibrio cholerae and is transmitted through contaminated water or food. Symptoms include profuse watery diarrhea, vomiting, leg cramps, and dehydration. In areas where medical help is scarce or unavailable, cholera can be deadly in a matter of hours if left untreated. The only way to prevent it is to take steps to ensure clean water and food sources.

The immune system response to cholera is complex. It begins with the production of antibodies specific for Vibrio cholerae, which triggers an inflammatory response in surrounding tissues. This inflammation helps keep the bacteria contained and prevents it from spreading throughout the body, allowing the immune system time to mount a more robust attack. The body may also produce proteins called interferons, which stimulate the activity of other immune system cells such as white blood cells and macrophages. These cells then engulf and digest any bacteria they come in contact with.

Cholera can be treated with antibiotics to kill the bacteria, and rehydration therapy to replace lost fluids and electrolytes. Vaccines may be given to those at risk of contracting the disease, such as travelers or people living in areas with poor access to safe water and sanitation. Proper handwashing, food preparation, and storage are also important for preventing the spread of cholera. In addition, educational campaigns can help raise awareness about proper hygiene measures that can reduce the risk of infection.

How Does Cholera Affect The Immune System?

Cholera infection triggers an immune system response, which is complex and involves multiple pathways. The initial defense is the production of antibodies against Vibrio cholerae which helps contain the bacteria in the local area and prevents it from spreading throughout the body. However, due to its fast-acting nature, this process may not be enough to completely eliminate the bacteria.

The body then activates other immune system cells such as white blood cells and macrophages to help fight the infection. These cells engulf and digest any bacteria they come in contact with, further helping to contain the infection. The body may also produce proteins called interferons which stimulate the activity of other immune system cells and spur them into action against the invading pathogen.

However, due to the extreme conditions of cholera infection, such as dehydration and electrolyte imbalance, the immune system may be weakened in its ability to respond effectively. It is therefore important to treat cholera with antibiotics and rehydration therapy in order to help restore balance and give the immune system a fighting chance against the pathogen.

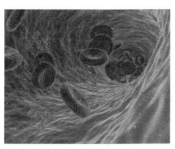

How Does One Develop Immunity Against Cholera?

Immunity to cholera can be developed through vaccination or natural exposure. Vaccines for cholera are available in certain areas where access to clean water and sanitation is limited, and they offer protection against the disease. Alternatively, individuals may gain immunity through natural exposure to the bacteria. This method has a much higher risk of severe illness or even death, however, so it is not recommended.

Another way to build immunity against cholera is through improved hygiene measures, such as proper handwashing and food preparation and storage. Educating individuals on these practices can help reduce the risk of infection and promote a healthier immune response to any future exposures. In addition, providing access to clean drinking water and proper sanitation facilities is essential for reducing cholera outbreaks in high-risk regions.

Tuberculosis

Tuberculosis (TB) is a highly contagious and potentially fatal bacterial infection caused by Mycobacterium tuberculosis. It affects the lungs primarily, but can also affect other organs such as the brain, spine, and kidneys. The infection is spread through close contact with an infected person or from droplets of their saliva or mucus when they cough, sneeze, or speak. Symptoms can include a persistent cough, fatigue, night sweats, shortness of breath, chest pain, and fever. If left untreated it can lead to serious health complications such as organ failure and death.

How Does Tuberculosis Affect The Immune System ?

Tuberculosis is a major challenge for the human immune system, due to its ability to evade and suppress host immunity. It can cause immunosuppression – weakening of natural defense mechanisms in the body which increases susceptibility to other infections. TB infection has been associated with an increased risk of HIV infection and other opportunistic infections such as cryptococcal meningitis or disseminated tuberculosis.

Infection with TB can also lead to the development of an abnormal immune response – known as a granulomatous reaction, whereby the body produces an excessive number of white blood cells in order to fight the infection. This causes inflammation and tissue damage, leading to symptoms such as weight loss and fever. Treatment typically includes antibiotics which are effective in controlling the spread of TB. However, complete control and prevention of TB is only possible with a strong and healthy immune system.

Therefore, it is important to ensure that your immune system is functioning properly by maintaining a balanced diet, exercising regularly, getting enough sleep, and avoiding stress as much as possible. Additionally, if you are at higher risk for TB such as healthcare workers, immunocompromised individuals, or those living in areas where TB is prevalent, it is recommended to get tested regularly for TB. With proper care and treatment, the effects of tuberculosis on your immune system can be minimized and its spread contained.

How Does One Develop Immunity Against Tuberculosis?

The human immune system has the ability to

develop protective immunity against tuberculosis when it is exposed to a controlled amount of bacteria. This is known as vaccination. Vaccines are available which can help protect individuals from TB infection and disease. The Bacillus Calmette-Guérin (BCG) vaccine is the only licensed vaccine available for the prevention of TB worldwide and has been in use since 1921. It is generally recommended for all children and adults who are at higher risk of TB infection or disease, such as healthcare workers, immunocompromised individuals, and those living in areas where TB is prevalent.

In addition to preventive vaccines, there are also treatments available which can help reduce the severity of symptoms associated with an active TB infection. These therapies typically involve a combination of drugs which target different aspects of the immune system, including the cells and molecules involved in the body's natural defenses against TB.

CHAPTER 6: AUTOIMMUNE DISEASES

Autoimmune diseases occur when the body's immune system mistakes healthy cells for foreign invaders and attacks them. This can lead to damage in various organs and tissues, such as the joints, skin, muscles, and blood vessels. Examples of autoimmune diseases include lupus, type 1 diabetes, multiple sclerosis (MS), rheumatoid arthritis (RA), psoriasis, and Graves' disease.

While the exact cause of autoimmune diseases is unknown, researchers believe that a combination of genetic, lifestyle, and environmental factors can increase an individual's risk. Treatment typically focuses on alleviating symptoms through medications such as corticosteroids, nonsteroidal anti-inflammatory drugs (NSAIDs), and immunosuppressants. Additionally, lifestyle changes such as eating a healthy diet and getting regular exercise may help manage the condition.

Type 1 Diabetes

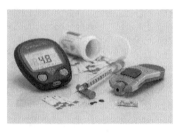

Type 1 diabetes occurs when the immune system attacks and destroys cells in the pancreas, specifically those that produce insulin. Insulin is a hormone needed to regulate blood sugar levels. Without enough insulin, glucose accumulates in the bloodstream, leading to type 1 diabetes. Symptoms of this condition include frequent urination, extreme thirst, hunger, fatigue, weight loss, irritability, and blurred vision.

Treatment for type 1 diabetes is focused on maintaining proper blood sugar levels through the use of insulin injections or an insulin pump. Additionally, lifestyle modifications such as eating a balanced diet, exercising regularly, and monitoring blood glucose levels can help manage the condition.

How Does Type 1 Diabetes Affect The Immune System ?

Type 1 diabetes is an autoimmune disorder that affects the functioning of the body's immune system. The body's immune system is responsible for recognizing and defending against foreign invaders, including viruses, bacteria, and other pathogens; however, in Type 1 Diabetes, the immune system mistakenly attacks and destroys healthy cells in the pancreas - specifically those that produce insulin - which is the hormone that helps regulate levels of glucose in the blood.

The exact cause of Type 1 Diabetes is still unknown; however, research has suggested a combination of genetic and environmental factors may be involved. Although diet and lifestyle changes can help manage symptoms of the disease, once it has developed there is no known cure or prevention strategy currently available.

How Does One Develop Immunity Against Type 1 Diabetes?

While there is currently no known cure for Type 1 Diabetes, scientists are researching ways to develop immunity against the autoimmune disorder. For instance, research has shown that certain types of cells derived from umbilical cord blood can be used as a potential treatment for Type 1 Diabetes. Additionally, various clinical trials and studies are being conducted around the world in an effort to discover more effective treatments and prevention strategies.

There are also lifestyle changes that those with Type 1 Diabetes can make in order to better manage the condition. For example, eating a balanced diet with plenty of fresh fruits and vegetables, exercising regularly and getting adequate sleep, and maintaining a healthy weight can help reduce symptoms associated with the disease. Additionally, it is important for people with Type 1 Diabetes to regularly monitor their blood sugar levels and take medications as prescribed by their doctor.

Multiple Sclerosis

Multiple sclerosis (MS) is a chronic autoimmune disease in which the immune system attacks the central nervous system, resulting in damage to the myelin sheaths surrounding nerve cells. Symptoms of MS vary depending on which nerves are affected and can include changes in sensation, muscle weakness, impaired coordination, vision problems, fatigue, and difficulty with balance.

Treatment for MS typically involves medications to reduce inflammation as well as medications to manage symptoms. Additionally, physical and occupational therapy can help with muscle weakness, coordination issues, and balance problems. Lifestyle modifications such as getting plenty of rest, eating a healthy diet, and reducing stress are also important for managing the condition.

How Multiple Sclerosis Affects The Immune System?

Multiple Sclerosis (MS) is an autoimmune disorder characterized by the immune system attacking its own healthy tissues. In this disorder, the body's T cells mistakenly attack myelin — a protective outer layer on nerve fibers — and can lead to inflammation of different parts of the central nervous system. This damage to myelin interferes with communication between nerve cells in the brain and spinal cord, leading to a wide variety of symptoms that vary greatly from patient to patient.

Unfortunately, MS has no known cure yet

but treatments can reduce its symptoms and slow disease progression. These treatments work by modulating the immune system and/ or reestablishing myelin production in certain areas. Immunomodulators suppress T-cell activity while interferons helps to reduce inflammation and regulate the immune system. In addition, glatiramer acetate is another drug that can be used to dampen the autoimmune response. Additionally, physical therapy can help with muscle weakness and other symptoms associated with MS.

How Does One Develop Immunity Against Multiple Sclerosis ?

Because MS is an autoimmune disorder, it cannot be prevented with traditional methods of immunization. However, there are some treatments that have been shown to reduce the risk of developing MS or slow its progression. These treatments include regular exercise and healthy dietary choices as well as managing stress levels. Studies also suggest that certain vitamins and supplements may help combat MS symptoms and promote overall health. Additionally, some research has shown that smoking may increase the risk of developing MS, so avoiding tobacco is recommended. Finally, it is important to get adequate rest each night and practice good hygiene since this can also help with managing stress levels and promoting overall health.

Rheumatoid Arthritis

Rheumatoid arthritis (RA) is a chronic autoimmune disorder that causes inflammation in the joints and other tissues. It occurs when the body's immune system attacks its own healthy cells, resulting in swelling, pain, and stiffness in the affected areas. Symptoms of RA can include fatigue, fever, loss of appetite, joint pain and swelling, and difficulty with everyday activities.

Treatment for RA typically involves medications to reduce inflammation as well as medications to manage symptoms. Additionally, physical and occupational therapy can help with muscle strength, flexibility, coordination issues, and balance problems. Lifestyle modifications such as eating a balanced diet and exercising regularly may also help manage the condition.

How Rheumatoid Arthritis Affects The Immune System?

Rheumatoid arthritis (RA) is an autoimmune disorder that affects the body's natural immune system. It causes inflammation of the joints and surrounding tissues, leading to pain, stiffness, swelling, and decreased mobility. The underlying cause of RA is not known, but it is thought to be triggered by a combination of genetic factors as well as environmental exposures such as infections, toxins, or trauma.

The immune system of a person with RA is

overactive and begins to attack healthy tissue in the body. This produces inflammatory molecules such as cytokines and chemokines which trigger inflammation and damage to the joints and surrounding tissues. As a result, the joint becomes inflamed, swollen, stiff and painful leading to decreased mobility. In addition, the inflammation can spread to other parts of the body such as the lungs, heart and other organs.

How Does One Develop Immunity Against Rheumatoid Arthritis ?

The primary goal of treating RA is to reduce inflammation and associated symptoms. The most common treatments are medications such as non-steroidal anti-inflammatory drugs (NSAIDs), corticosteroids, disease modifying antirheumatic drugs (DMARDs), and biologics. These medications help to suppress the immune system and reduce inflammation. It is also important to maintain a healthy lifestyle with regular exercise, good nutrition, and stress management.

Immune-based therapies are being explored as potential treatments for RA. One example is immunotherapy, which involves introducing small amounts of an antigen or causative agent to the body in order to induce an immune response that can protect against autoimmune diseases such as RA. Research is also looking into the use of probiotics and other natural products to modulate the immune system and reduce inflammation.

Lupus

Lupus is a chronic autoimmune disorder, meaning it occurs when the immune system mistakenly attacks healthy tissue. It can affect the skin, joints, and organs such as the kidneys, heart, and lungs. Common symptoms of lupus include fatigue, joint pain or swelling, skin rashes, fever, chest pain during deep breaths (pleurisy), hair loss, and anemia.

How Does Lupus Affect The Immune System?

When someone has lupus, their immune system produces antibodies (autoantibodies) that mistakenly attack healthy tissue instead of attacking foreign invaders like viruses or bacteria. This can cause inflammation in various parts of the body, which can lead to pain, swelling, and other symptoms. In addition, lupus can lead to a decrease in immune system function and an increased risk for infections. Treatment typically involves medications that reduce inflammation and suppress the immune system, allowing the body to heal itself.

What Are The Long-Term Effects Of Lupus On The Immune System?

The long-term effects of lupus on the immune system depend largely on how quickly and effectively a person is able to manage the condition. Over time, prolonged inflammation caused by lupus can lead to organ damage and other complications such as kidney failure, stroke, heart disease, and even death. Early diagnosis and treatment are important in managing lupus and helping people maintain healthy immune systems for as long as possible.

How Does One Develop Immunity Against Lupus?

Although there is no known way to develop immunity against lupus, early detection and treatment are the best ways to reduce inflammation and keep the immune system as healthy as possible. Treatment typically involves medications such as corticosteroids or immunosuppressants that can help reduce inflammation and suppress the immune system. Additionally, lifestyle modifications such as eating a well-balanced diet, getting regular exercise, and avoiding triggers such as stress, ultraviolet light exposure, and certain medications can reduce the risk of flares. Taking these steps can help people with lupus maintain a healthy immune system and reduce their risk of complications.

Inflammatory Bowel Disease

Inflammatory Bowel Disease (IBD) is an umbrella term for a group of chronic disorders that cause inflammation in the digestive tract. Common symptoms of IBD include abdominal pain, cramping, diarrhea, and rectal bleeding. IBD can affect both the small and large intestine and is typically treated with medications such as anti-inflammatory drugs or immunosuppressants that suppress the immune system.

How Does IBD Affect The Immune System?

In individuals with IBD, the immune system becomes overactive and attacks healthy tissue in the digestive tract. This leads to inflammation and irritation of the lining of the intestine, causing symptoms such as abdominal pain and diarrhea. The inflammation caused by IBD can also lead to a decrease in immune system function and an increased risk for infections.

What Are The Long-Term Effects Of IBD On The Immune System?

The long-term effects of IBD on the immune system depend largely on how quickly and effectively a person is able to manage the condition. Over time, prolonged inflammation caused by IBD can lead to organ damage and other complications such as malnutrition, anemia, and even cancer. Early diagnosis and treatment are important in managing IBD and helping people maintain healthy immune systems for as long as possible.

How Does One Develop Immunity Against IBD?

Unfortunately, there is no known way to develop immunity against IBD. However, early detection and treatment are the best ways to reduce inflammation and keep the immune system as healthy as possible. Treatment typically involves medications such as corticosteroids or immunosuppressants that can help reduce inflammation and suppress the immune system. Additionally, lifestyle modifications such as eating a well-balanced diet, getting regular exercise, and avoiding triggers such as stress, smoking, and certain medications can reduce the risk of flares. Taking these steps can help people with IBD maintain a healthy immune system and reduce their risk of complications.

Psoriasis

Psoriasis is a chronic autoimmune disorder in which the body's immune system attacks healthy skin cells. This results in patches of thick, scaly skin that are red and itchy. Psoriasis can affect any part of the body, but most commonly affects the elbows, knees, scalp, and lower back.

How Psoriasis Affects The Immune System?

Psoriasis is a chronic autoimmune disease that affects the skin and causes it to become red, inflamed, and scaly. It is thought to be caused by an overactive immune system that mistakenly attacks healthy skin cells. When this happens, the skin's natural response is to produce more cells than usual, causing thick patches of raised skin known as plaques.

These plaques are usually found on the elbows,

knees, scalp, and lower back. In addition to the physical symptoms of psoriasis, it can also cause emotional distress due to its appearance and symptom flare-ups.

The underlying cause of psoriasis is not fully understood yet but researchers believe that it is linked to an overactive immune system. In people with psoriasis, the immune system mistakenly attacks healthy skin cells and triggers an inflammatory response. This causes the body to produce more skin cells than normal, leading to thick plaques of raised skin.

The exact mechanism behind this is still unclear but experts believe it involves a combination of genetic factors and environmental triggers such as stress, infection, certain medications, or even sunburns.

The immune system plays an important role in controlling flares of psoriasis. When the body is exposed to certain triggers, the immune system becomes overactive and sends signals that cause inflammation and increased skin cell production. Treatments for psoriasis aim to reduce this activity by suppressing the immune system or targeting specific inflammatory pathways.

How Does One Develop Immunity Against Psoriasis?

Developing immunity against psoriasis is a complex process and it involves understanding the underlying causes of the disease. For example, some people may be genetically predisposed to the condition, which means that they are more likely to develop the condition if exposed to certain triggers such as stress or infections.

There is no single "cure" for psoriasis, but there are treatments that can help manage symptoms and reduce flares. Treatment options range from topical medications to systemic immunosuppressants. These treatments work by targeting the underlying cause of psoriasis, which is an overactive immune system.

In some cases, lifestyle changes may also help reduce flares and improve overall health. Eating a balanced diet, reducing stress, and avoiding triggers such as smoking or alcohol can all help to reduce flares of psoriasis. Regular exercise has also been shown to be beneficial for people with psoriasis, as it can improve overall health and wellbeing.

Developing immunity against psoriasis is a complex process that involves understanding the underlying cause of the disease and finding the right treatment plan for the individual. In addition to medical treatments, lifestyle changes and avoiding known triggers can also help reduce flares and improve overall wellbeing.

What Are Some Of The Long-Term Implications?

Psoriasis is a chronic condition that has the

potential to impact one's life in many ways. Some of these impacts include physical discomfort due to the itching, pain, and inflammation associated with psoriasis. In addition, psychological effects such as depression, anxiety, and low self-esteem can also occur due to the visible changes in skin appearance.

Long-term complications of psoriasis may include joint damage from arthritis caused by chronic inflammation of joints in the body. This type of joint damage is known as psoriatic arthritis and can lead to permanent joint damage if untreated. Psoriasis can also increase the risk of certain conditions such as metabolic syndrome, cardiovascular disease, and type 2 diabetes.

It is important to take proactive steps to manage psoriasis in order to reduce the potential long-term implications. This includes following a treatment plan that works best for the individual and being aware of any changes in symptoms that could indicate a flare. In addition, living a healthy lifestyle with regular exercise, eating a balanced diet, and reducing stress can help reduce flares and improve overall wellbeing.

By understanding how psoriasis affects the immune system and taking proactive steps to manage it, individuals can minimize its long-term complications. With the right treatment plan and lifestyle adjustments, it is possible to reduce flares and improve quality of life for those living with psoriasis.

Graves' Disease

Graves' disease is an autoimmune disorder in which the body's immune system attacks healthy cells in the thyroid gland, leading to over-production of hormones. Symptoms of Graves' disease can include fatigue, a fast heartbeat, weight loss, tremors, and bulging eyes.

Treatment for Graves' disease typically involves medications to reduce hormone production as well as medications to manage symptoms. Additionally, lifestyle modifications such as eating a balanced diet and reducing stress can help manage the condition. Surgery may also be necessary in more severe cases.

How Graves' Disease Affect The Immune System?

Graves' disease is an autoimmune disorder that affects the thyroid gland. It causes the body's immune system to attack healthy tissue, leading to symptoms such as fatigue, muscle weakness, weight gain, and depression. In some cases, Graves' disease can cause changes in the eyes which can lead to vision problems.

The exact cause of Graves' disease is unknown, but it is believed to be caused by a combination of genetic and environmental factors. It is more common in women than men and tends to run in families.

When the immune system detects something that it considers a threat, it will produce antibodies to fight off the invader. In people with Graves' disease, the immune system mistakenly identifies healthy tissue as a potential threat and produces antibodies that attack the thyroid gland. This causes inflammation which can lead to symptoms such as an enlarged thyroid, fatigue, irregular heart beat, and weight gain.

How Does One Develop Immunity Against Graves' Disease?

Unfortunately, since the cause of Graves' disease is unknown, there is no known way to prevent its development. However, managing stress levels and getting enough rest can help reduce your risk of developing the disorder. It may also be beneficial to get tested for any underlying autoimmune conditions that may be contributing to your symptoms. Additionally, eating a healthy diet and exercising regularly can help support a healthy immune system and reduce your risk of developing Graves' disease.

Since Graves' disease is an autoimmune condition, treatments focus on suppressing the overactive immune response. This may involve medications such as corticosteroids or immunosuppressants. In some cases, radiation therapy or surgery may be used to remove part of the thyroid gland. Alternative treatments such as acupuncture or homeopathic remedies may also be beneficial.

It is important to talk to your doctor about the best treatment option for you, as every case of Graves' disease is unique and requires a personalized approach. With proper treatment, many people with Graves' disease can manage their symptoms and live full lives.

What Are The Long-Term Effects Of Graves' Disease On The Immune System?

The long term effects of Graves' disease on the immune system depend largely on how it is treated. If left untreated, the damage to the thyroid can lead to complications such as hypothyroidism or goiter. Additionally, untreated Graves' disease can increase a person's risk for developing other autoimmune disorders or infections.

When Graves' disease is treated, the goal is to restore balance in the immune system. While this usually results in a reduced risk of complications, it also means that the body is less able to fight off infections or other invaders. Therefore, people with Graves' disease should take extra precautions to stay healthy and avoid infection whenever possible. Additionally, regular checkups with a doctor can help monitor for any potential complications.

With proper treatment and care, many people with Graves' disease are able to manage their symptoms and live healthy lives. It is important to talk to your doctor about the best ways to support your immune system and reduce your risk of further complications.

Age-Related Changes To Immunity

As we age, our immune system undergoes changes that can lead to an increased susceptibility to certain types of infections. One of the most common age-related changes is a decrease in the number and activity of the white blood cells that help fight off infectious agents. In addition, age-related changes may also produce a decrease in antibodies which may reduce the body's ability to respond to new pathogens. As a result, the elderly may often be more susceptible to influenza and pneumonia than younger people.

To help protect against age-related changes in immunity, it is important for older adults to stay up-to-date on their vaccinations. Vaccines can provide protection from specific illnesses like flu or pneumococcal disease, as well as help to boost the body's natural immunity. Additionally, they may be able to prevent serious illnesses and complications that can result from having a weakened immune system. Regular health screenings and tests are also important for monitoring changes in the immune system and for treating any infections that do occur.

In addition to vaccinations and regular health screenings, there are other measures that older adults can take to stay healthy. Adequate nutrition, exercise, and rest are all key components of a strong immune system. Eating a balanced diet with plenty of fresh fruits and vegetables is essential for the body's ability to fight off infections. Exercise not only helps strengthen the muscles and bones, but also strengthens the immune system by increasing circulation of white blood cells throughout the body. Finally, adequate rest is critical for the body to fight off infections and recover from illness. Taking these measures can help seniors maintain a healthy immune system as they age.

Finally, it is important to be aware of the signs and symptoms of infection. Early detection and treatment can help prevent serious complications from any illness. Knowing the signs and symptoms of infection, as well as what steps to take if they occur, can also make seniors more prepared in the event that they contract an illness or infection due to their weakened immune system.

CHAPTER 7 : ALLERGIES AND INFECTIOUS DISEASES

Allergies are an immune system response to harmless substances that can cause uncomfortable symptoms. The human immune system is made up of a number of cells, tissues, and organs that work together to protect against foreign invaders like viruses or bacteria. When these allergens enter your body, your immune system recognizes them as something it doesn't recognize and produces antibodies to fight off the foreign substance.

When these allergens are encountered again, the body responds by producing an excessive amount of antibodies which can lead to allergies like hay fever or skin rashes. Common allergens include pollen, dust mites, mold spores, pet dander, and certain foods. To avoid allergic reactions, it is important to reduce your exposure to known allergens and avoid triggering factors.

Types Of Allergies

Allergies are divided into two types: seasonal allergies or hay fever, and perennial allergies.

Seasonal Allergies

Seasonal allergies, also known as hay fever, are a response of the immune system to allergens present in the environment at specific times of the year. These allergens could include pollen from trees, grass, and weeds, which are typically prevalent in the spring, summer, or fall seasons. Symptoms of seasonal allergies can range from mild to severe and may include sneezing, runny or stuffy nose, itchy or watery eyes, and itchy throat or ears.

Perennial Allergies

Perennial allergies, unlike seasonal allergies, can occur throughout the year. The immune system reacts to allergens that are typically present in the environment regardless of the season. Common triggers for perennial allergies include dust mites, pet dander, mold, and cockroaches. Symptoms are similar to seasonal allergies and can include sneezing, runny or stuffy nose, itchy or watery eyes, and itchy throat. Despite the constant potential exposure to these allergens, the severity of symptoms can vary from person to person and may be managed with the proper medication and environmental control measures.

Common Items That Can Trigger Allergic Reactions

The immune system is the body's natural protection against foreign invaders, but sometimes it can get confused and launch an attack on something harmless like pet fur or pollen. This type of reaction is called an allergy, and it happens when your immune system overreacts to a substance that's usually harmless to most people.

Common items that can trigger allergic reactions include pollen, pet fur, dust mites, mold spores, certain foods and even insect stings. Allergens can exist both indoors and outdoors, and exposure to them can cause a variety of symptoms including coughing, sneezing, runny nose, watery eyes and even rashes or hives.

pollen is one of the most common allergens. Pollen particles are released by plants, and they can irritate the eyes, nose and throat when inhaled. Common seasonal allergies to watch out for include ragweed, grasses and tree pollen.

Pet fur can also cause an allergic reaction in some people. This type of allergy is caused by proteins that cats and dogs release into the air. Symptoms of a pet fur allergy may include sneezing, itchy eyes or skin rashes.

Dust mites are tiny bugs commonly found in bedding, carpets and furniture. They feed off of dead skin cells, and their excrement can cause allergic reactions such as asthma attacks or wheezing.

Mold spores can also be a big problem for people with allergies. Mold is often found in damp or humid environments, and it can trigger asthma attacks as well as other types of allergic reactions.

Certain foods can also cause an allergic reaction. These include eggs, dairy products, nuts, shellfish and wheat. Eating even small amounts of these foods can cause anaphylaxis – a life-threatening reaction that requires immediate medical attention.

Insect stings can also cause an allergic reaction in some people. Symptoms of this type of allergy may include hives, itching and swelling. In severe cases, anaphylaxis can occur due to an insect sting allergy.

Allergies And The Immune System

Allergies are a common disorder that affect the immune system. When an individual is exposed to something they are allergic to, their body mounts an immune response. This response can include sneezing, coughing, itchy eyes, runny nose, hives, and in some cases severe difficulty breathing or even anaphylaxis.

At the heart of an allergic response is a type of white blood cell known as a mast cell, which releases histamine in the presence of allergens. Histamine triggers an inflammatory response from other cells, and this causes the typical symptoms of allergies. People with allergies have mast cells that are overly sensitive to certain substances – for example, pollen or dust mites – and react even when there is no real threat.

The exact cause of allergies is not completely understood, but it is believed to involve a combination of genetic and environmental factors. Allergies can be managed with lifestyle changes, diet modifications, and medications. Immunotherapy may also be recommended for some patients in order to desensitize the immune system to the allergen. Immunotherapy works by introducing small amounts of the allergen to the body over time so that it becomes less reactive and more tolerant.

The Development Of Asthma And Allergies

It is believed that genetics play a role in the development of asthma and allergies. However, environmental factors can also be a contributing factor to the development of these conditions. Allergens from dust mites, pet dander, cockroaches, mold spores, and pollen are some common triggers for people with allergies or asthma.

When these triggers are present, a person's immune system can overreact and cause inflammation of the airways leading to asthma attacks or even anaphylaxis. This is why it is so important to be aware of environmental triggers and take precautions when possible to limit exposure.

In addition, allergies can also be developed from food or medications that trigger a reaction in a person's immune system. Common food allergies include nuts, dairy, shellfish, and eggs. It is also possible to develop an allergy to a medication over time if it triggers an immune response in the body.

These conditions can be managed with medications or lifestyle changes depending on the severity of the condition and individual needs. Taking steps to minimize exposure to allergens can help reduce symptoms and improve quality of life. If you have questions or concerns, speak with your healthcare provider to find the best treatment for you.

Infectious Diseases

The immune system is a network of cells, tissues, and organs that work together to protect the body from disease-causing microorganisms. When faced with an infectious agent, such as a virus or bacteria, the immune system responds by producing antibodies to fight the invader. The presence of these antibodies helps the body recognize foreign substances and initiate an immune response to protect against the infection.

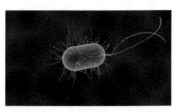

Bacteria

Bacteria are microscopic organisms that can cause a variety of diseases. They can be found almost everywhere in the environment, and some types of bacteria are beneficial for us. However, many species of bacteria are considered harmful to humans because they can cause infections such as pneumonia, meningitis, gonorrhea, and strep throat. By understanding more about these microscopic pathogens, we can better protect ourselves and our loved ones from infection.

In the body, bacteria can be both beneficial and harmful. Beneficial bacteria help keep our digestive system functioning properly by breaking down food and producing vitamins that our bodies cannot make on their own. These bacteria also help to strengthen our immune systems against invading disease-causing organisms such as viruses and fungi.

When harmful bacteria enter the body, they can cause a range of illnesses from mild to severe. They can also be spread from person to person through contact with saliva or other bodily fluids such as blood and vomit. It's important to practice good hygiene by washing your hands regularly, using face masks when necessary, and avoiding contact with people who are visibly sick.

Types Of Bacteria

Bacteria come in many varieties. Some common examples include Escherichia coli (E. coli), Salmonella, Staphylococcus aureus (staph), Klebsiella pneumonia, and Clostridium difficile (C. diff). Each type of bacteria has its own set of characteristics that make it unique from other bacteria.

The majority of bacterial infections are caused by Gram-positive bacteria, which have a thicker cell wall than Gram-negative bacteria. These types of bacteria can be treated with antibiotics and other medications, depending on the severity of the infection. On the other hand, some species of Gram-positive and Gram-negative bacteria are resistant to many commonly used antibiotics.

Other types of bacteria can cause more serious infections, such as meningitis and sepsis. These bacteria are typically treated with stronger antibiotics or antiviral medications, which target the specific type of infection that is present. In some cases, these infections may require hospitalization or even surgery to effectively treat them.

How Do Bacteria Affect The Immune System?

The immune system is your body's natural defense against infection. When a harmful bacteria or virus enters the body, the immune system identifies it and sends out an army of white blood cells to fight off the invader. The cells help to destroy invading organisms by producing antibodies that recognize and bind to them.

When the immune system is functioning properly, it can help keep harmful bacteria and viruses at bay. However, when the immune system is weak or compromised, it can be more difficult for the body to fight off these invading organisms, leading to a greater risk of infection.

Certain medical conditions can also put individuals at higher risk for infections because they weaken the immune system. These include chemotherapy, HIV/AIDS, diabetes, and autoimmune diseases. People with weakened immune systems should take extra precautions to prevent infection by avoiding contact with those who are ill and practicing good hygiene.

Immunizations also help strengthen the immune system against certain types of bacteria and viruses, making it easier for the body to fight off these invaders if they do enter the body. Vaccines contain a weakened form of an infectious organism, which is injected into the body to stimulate the immune system and help it build up immunity against that particular pathogen.

Viruses

Viruses are small microscopic organisms that can cause disease in humans, animals and plants. They are composed of genetic material (DNA or RNA) surrounded by a protective coat called a capsid. Viruses only reproduce within the cells of other living organisms, meaning they cannot reproduce on their own.

When viruses come into contact with healthy cells, they attach themselves to the cells and inject their genetic material. This causes the genes of the virus to be replicated, as well as interfering with the normal functioning of the cell. These changes can cause a variety of symptoms, including fever, tiredness, headache or even organ failure if left untreated.

Fortunately, our bodies have an amazing defense system that fights off most viruses before they can cause any harm. The immune system is made up of white blood cells, antibodies and other organs which identify viruses, target them and eliminate them from the body. Vaccines are also used to protect against certain infectious diseases by stimulating the body's own immune response.

Types Of Viruses

Viruses come in a variety of shapes and sizes. The most common type is the RNA virus, which contains only one strand of genetic material that it uses to replicate itself. Other viral families include DNA viruses, retroviruses, orthomyxoviruses (which cause flu-like illnesses) and adenoviruses (which can cause respiratory infections).

Viruses are also classified according to which host they infect - animals, humans or plants. Some viruses, such as the common cold virus, can infect both humans and animals while others are specific to one species.

No matter what type of virus it is, the immune system's response is always the same: to target and eliminate it from the body. By understanding how viruses work and how our immune systems protect us from them, we can better protect ourselves against infection.

How Do Viruses Affect The Immune System?

The immune system plays a crucial role in protecting us from viruses and other pathogens. When the body is exposed to a virus, the immune system rapidly produces cells that can recognize and destroy it. This process is called the adaptive immune response.

When the immune system recognizes a virus, it triggers an inflammatory response. This activates white blood cells (such as T-cells and B-cells) to produce antibodies, which attach to the virus and prevent it from infecting other cells. The body also releases proteins called cytokines that help control inflammation.

The immune system can also remember past infections, enabling it to recognize a virus more quickly the next time it is exposed. This is why vaccinations are so effective - they teach our bodies how to recognize and fight off a certain virus quickly and efficiently.

The immune system is an amazing defense system that helps us stay healthy, but it can also be weakened by factors such as poor nutrition, stress or lack of sleep. When our immune systems are not functioning properly, we are more vulnerable to viral infections. That's why it's important to take care of our bodies and give our immune systems the support they need to keep us healthy.

What Is The Meaning Of Fungi ?

The term fungi refers to a group of eukaryotic organisms that includes yeasts, molds, and mushrooms. Fungi are typically found in damp environments and feed on organic material. They can cause diseases of plants, animals, and humans by invading tissues or entering the bloodstream via open wounds. In terms of the immune system, fungi can stimulate an inflammatory response and produce toxins that can damage host tissues. Some species of fungi also produce antigens, which allow them to be recognized by the immune system, resulting in a heightened immune response. Fungi are among the most common causes of infectious disease. Treatment typically involves antifungal medications and supportive care.

Types Of Fungi

Fungi can be classified into three major groups: zygomycetes, ascomycetes, and basidiomycetes. Zygomycetes are fungi that reproduce via the formation of asexual spores. Examples include black bread mold and Rhizopus species. Ascomycetes are fungi that reproduce via the formation of sexual spores. Examples include yeasts (e.g., Saccharomyces species) and molds (e.g., Penicillium species). Basidiomycetes are fungi that reproduce via the formation of basidiospores, which are produced by specialized structures called basidia. Examples include mushrooms (e.g., Agaricus species) and puffballs (e.g., Calvatia species).

Effects Of Fungi On The Immune System

Fungi can cause a variety of illnesses, from skin infections to life-threatening systemic diseases. The immune system plays a critical role in defending against fungal infections by identifying antigens and producing antibodies to neutralize the infective organisms. In some cases, however, fungal infections can overstimulate the immune system, leading to a condition known as chronic hypersensitivity pneumonitis or "fungal asthma". This is an inflammatory lung disorder caused by inhalation of fungal spores and antigens. Treatment typically involves medications to control inflammation and eliminate the infection.

Prevention Of Fungal Infections

The best way to prevent fungal infections is to practice good hygiene and keep the environment clean. In addition, wearing protective clothing and avoiding contact with potentially contaminated surfaces can also reduce the risk of infection. Vaccines are available for certain types of fungi, such as Cryptococcus neoformans, which can help prevent serious illness. Finally, antifungal medications can be used to treat and prevent fungal infections.

Fungal diseases are a common cause of infectious disease, but with proper prevention and treatment they can often be managed successfully. By understanding the role fungi play in the immune system, we can better protect ourselves from harm and improve our overall health.

HIV

Human immunodeficiency virus (HIV) is a viral infection that attacks the body's immune system, making it less able to fight off other infections and diseases. HIV is spread through contact with infected bodily fluids, such as blood or semen. If left untreated, HIV can lead to acquired immunodeficiency syndrome (AIDS), which is the most advanced stage of HIV infection. Early diagnosis and treatment are essential for controlling the virus and preventing progression to AIDS. Treatment typically involves antiretroviral therapy, which is a combination of medications that suppress the virus and prevent it from replicating. It is important to follow up with regular testing to monitor progress and ensure treatment is effective. HIV/AIDS continues to be a major public health concern, particularly in low-income countries. Prevention efforts focus on increasing access to testing and treatment, as well as reducing behaviours that increase the risk of infection.

How Does Hiv Affect The Immune System ?

HIV infects and destroys CD4+ T cells, which play a major role in the body's adaptive immune response. As more CD4+ cells are destroyed, the immune system becomes weakened and is unable to efficiently fight off other infections or diseases. This can lead to opportunistic infections, such as candidiasis (yeast infection), pneumocystis pneumonia, and tuberculosis. HIV also increases the risk of certain types of cancer, including Kaposi's sarcoma and non-Hodgkin's lymphoma. Antiretroviral therapy can help restore the immune system and reduce the risk of opportunistic infections and cancer, but it is important to continue treatment even after symptoms improve.

AIDS

Acquired immunodeficiency syndrome (AIDS) is the most advanced stage of HIV infection. It is characterized by a weakened immune system, which leaves the body unable to fight off other infections and diseases. AIDS develops when a person's CD4+ T cell count drops below 200 cells/mm3 or when they develop an opportunistic infection. Treatment typically involves antiretroviral therapy to suppress the virus and prevent it from replicating. It is important to follow up with regular testing to monitor progress and ensure treatment is effective. Prevention efforts focus on increasing access to testing, treatment, and education about safe behaviours that reduce the risk of HIV transmission.

While there is currently no cure for AIDS, treatments are available to help control the virus and prevent progression to AIDS. By understanding how HIV affects the immune system, we can work together to promote prevention, testing, treatment, and support for those living with HIV/AIDS.

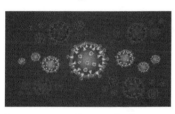

How Does Aids Affect The Immune System ?

AIDS is the most advanced stage of HIV infection, characterized by a weakened immune system. As a result, people living with AIDS are more susceptible to opportunistic infections and other illnesses. This is because their bodies are unable to effectively fight off pathogens due to the destruction of important immune cells such as CD4+ T cells. Treatment typically involves antiretroviral therapy to suppress the virus and prevent it from replicating. It is important to follow up with regular testing to monitor progress and ensure treatment is effective. Prevention efforts focus on increasing access to testing, treatment, and education about safe behaviours that reduce the risk of HIV transmission.

By understanding how AIDS affects the immune system, we can work together to promote prevention, testing, treatment, and support for those living with HIV/AIDS. With proper medical care, people living with AIDS can lead long and healthy lives.

Immune Deficiencies

Immune deficiencies are conditions that occur when the immune system is not working properly. When your immune system is weak, it's less able to fight off disease and infection. Immune deficiencies can be caused by medical treatments like chemotherapy or radiation, certain medicines and genetic disorders. They can also develop if part of the body's normal immune system isn't functioning properly, due to a virus or other infection.

Some of the most common types of immune deficiency include:

What Is The Meaning Of Hypogammaglobulinemia?

Hypogammaglobulinemia is a condition that occurs when the body's level of antibodies, or gamma globulin, is very low. When this happens, the body becomes more susceptible to infections and other illnesses because it cannot fight off invading organisms as effectively. This condition can be caused by a variety of factors such as certain medications or an underlying medical condition.

It is often treated with immunoglobulin replacement therapy, which boosts the body's ability to fight off infections. In some cases, lifestyle changes and improved nutrition can also help manage this condition.

How Does Hypogammaglobulinemia Affect The Immune System ?

Hypogammaglobulinemia affects the immune system by reducing the ability of the body's immune cells to fight off infections and other illnesses. Without adequate numbers of antibodies, the body is unable to mount an effective response against invading organisms or environmental toxins. This can lead to frequent and more severe forms of infection, including bacterial and viral diseases. Additionally, individuals with Hypogammaglobulinemia are at increased risk for certain cancers and autoimmune diseases.

How Is Hypogammaglobulinemia Treated?

Hypogammaglobulinemia is typically treated through immunoglobulin replacement therapy, which involves receiving a regular infusion of concentrated antibodies. This helps to boost the body's ability to fight off infection and can be used in combination with other treatments such as antibiotics or antivirals. In some cases, lifestyle changes may also help to keep the condition under control, including eating a balanced diet, engaging in regular exercise, and avoiding alcohol and smoking. Additionally, keeping up with regular doctor visits is important for ongoing monitoring of the condition.

It is important to note that everyone's condition and treatment plan will be different, so it is best to speak with your doctor about the best approach for managing Hypogammaglobulinemia.

Are There Any Complications Associated With Hypogammaglobulinemia?

Yes, there are a few potential complications associated with Hypogammaglobulinemia. These include an increased risk of infections and cancer, as well as an increased susceptibility to autoimmune diseases. Additionally, individuals with this condition may be at greater risk for developing sepsis, a potentially life-threatening complication caused by a severe infection. It is important to talk to your doctor about the potential risks and benefits associated with your treatment plan in order to minimize the potential for complications.

By understanding and managing Hypogammaglobulinemia, individuals can be better equipped to fight off infection and maintain good health. It is important to work with your doctor to form an individualized treatment plan that is right for you. With proper management, living with Hypogammaglobulinemia can be manageable and even enjoyable.

What Is The Meaning Of Severe Combined Immunodeficiency ?

Severe Combined Immunodeficiency (SCID) is a rare, inherited disorder of the immune system. Individuals with SCID lack both T- and B-lymphocyte functioning, which results in an inability to fight infections and other illnesses. This makes it difficult for the body to recover from even minor infections or injuries. Without proper treatment, individuals with SCID usually do not live to adulthood.

How Does Severe Combined Immunodeficiency Affect The Immune System ?

Severe Combined Immunodeficiency (SCID) affects the immune system by reducing or eliminating the body's ability to fight off infections and other illnesses. Without adequate numbers of functioning immune cells, the body lacks the ability to mount an effective response against invading organisms or environmental toxins. This can lead to frequent and more severe forms of infection, including bacterial and viral diseases. Additionally, individuals with SCID are at increased risk for certain cancers and autoimmune diseases.

It is important to note that the effects of SCID on the immune system vary by individual, so it is best to speak with your doctor about your specific condition. By understanding and managing SCID, individuals can be better equipped to fight off infection and maintain good health. It is important to work with your doctor to form an individualized treatment plan that is right for you.

How Is Severe Combined Immunodeficiency Treated?

Severe Combined Immunodeficiency (SCID) is typically treated with a bone marrow transplant, which replaces the damaged or missing immune cells with healthy ones from a donor. This helps restore the body's ability to fight off infection and other illnesses. Additionally, some individuals may receive immunoglobulin replacement therapy to boost their immune system's response to invading organisms. In some cases, lifestyle changes such as eating a healthy diet and exercising regularly can also help manage SCID symptoms. It is important to speak with your doctor about the best treatment plan for you.

Are There Any Complications Associated With Severe Combined Immunodeficiency ?

Yes, individuals with SCID may be at an increased risk for complications such as cancer and infection. Additionally, some individuals may experience long-term health effects from the bone marrow transplant and immunoglobulin replacement therapies used to treat this condition. It is important to talk to your doctor about the potential risks and benefits associated with your treatment plan in order to minimize the potential for complications.

By understanding Severe Combined Immunodeficiency (SCID) and its associated treatments, individuals can be better equipped to maintain their health. It is important to work with your doctor to form an individualized treatment plan that is right for you.

CHAPTER 8: VACCINES
AND BEYOND

Immunology is a fascinating field of science that explores the ways in which our bodies protect themselves from disease. Vaccines are the most well-known application of immunology, but there are many more potential applications just waiting to be explored.

One area that has seen tremendous growth in recent years is immunotherapies. Immunotherapies are treatments that use the body's natural immune system to fight diseases such as cancer in ways that traditional treatments can't. By harnessing the power of the immune system, these therapies can provide hope for even those who have been given up on by conventional medicine.

Another application being explored is gene therapy. This involves using genetic information to treat diseases at the source. By altering a patient's genetic code in specific ways, it is possible to target particular types of diseases and even create treatments for those who have not responded to traditional therapies.

What Are The Types Of Vaccines?

Vaccines can be broadly classified according to four types: inactivated vaccines, live attenuated

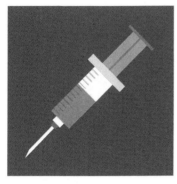 vaccines, subunit vaccines, and toxoid vaccines.

Inactivated Vaccines are made from a weakened version of the pathogen that has been killed using physical or chemical means. Examples of inactivated vaccines include the flu shot and the polio vaccine.

Live Attenuated Vaccines are made from a weakened or altered version of the pathogen or virus that is still alive. Examples of live attenuated vaccines include the measles, mumps, and rubella (MMR) vaccine and the chickenpox vaccine.

Subunit Vaccines are made from components of the disease-causing microorganism such as proteins, carbohydrates, or toxins. Examples of subunit vaccines include the hepatitis B vaccine and the human papillomavirus (HPV) vaccine.

Toxoid Vaccines are made from inactivated toxin produced by certain bacteria. An example of a toxoid vaccine is the diphtheria/tetanus/pertussis (DTP) vaccine.

1.Live Attenuated Vaccines

Live attenuated vaccines contain a weakened version of the pathogen that causes the disease.

Once administered, these weakened pathogens cause an infection in the body which triggers an immune response from the recipient. The recipient's own white blood cells and antibodies will then respond to this weakened pathogen, ultimately leading to immunity against more infectious forms of the same virus or bacteria. Live attenuated vaccines are some of the most effective vaccination agents out there since they generate robust immune responses that last for long periods of time. Due to this, live attenuated vaccines are used to protect against several diseases such as measles, mumps, rubella and yellow fever. Though these types of vaccines can be very effective in preventing disease from occurring in a patient, they may carry a slight risk of the weakened virus or bacteria reverting to its full-fledged pathogenic form. As such, it is important for people being vaccinated with live attenuated vaccines to take extra caution in their hygiene practices and heeding medical advice during their immunization.

What Is The Chemical Reaction That Occurs In The Immune System?

The chemical reaction that occurs when a live attenuated vaccine is administered to an individual is twofold. First, the weakened pathogen stimulates the body's immune system by triggering it to create and produce antibodies specific to that particular virus or bacteria. These antibodies then attach themselves onto white blood cells, such as neutrophils, lymphocytes and macrophages, and fight off the weakened virus or bacteria. As a result of this reaction, the body develops a memory of the pathogen so that it can quickly recognize it should an infection occur in future. This is how vaccines ultimately provide immunity against more infectious forms of the same virus or bacteria.

Another chemical reaction that occurs when a live attenuated vaccine is administered is cytokine production. Cytokines are proteins released by cells of the immune system that act as messengers and help to regulate the body's response to infection or inflammation. In the case of live attenuated vaccines, cytokines play a crucial role in helping to activate other cells of the immune system such as memory B and T cells, which are essential for mounting a defense against an infection.

2. Subunit Vaccines

Subunit vaccines are made up of components of the pathogen, such as proteins or toxins, that have been isolated from the virus or bacteria itself. These components are then combined with other substances in order to form a vaccine and produce an immune response in the recipient. Subunit vaccines do not contain any live pathogens but instead rely on the body's own immune system to recognize the specific components of the pathogen and generate a response. Unlike live attenuated vaccines, these types of vaccines do not pose the risk of reverting back into their full-fledged form since it does not contain any living pathogens. However, subunit vaccines are generally less effective than live attenuated vaccines since they may not be able to stimulate a strong enough immune response in the recipient. Subunit vaccines are typically used to protect against diseases such as influenza, hepatitis B and whooping cough.

What Is The Chemical Reaction That Occurs In The Immune System?

The chemical reaction that occurs when a subunit vaccine is administered to an individual is similar to live attenuated vaccines in that antibodies specific to the virus or bacteria are produced. The difference lies in the fact that the antibodies are generated by the body's own immune system and not from a live pathogen. When the vaccine components enter the body, they stimulate white blood cells, such as B-cells and T-cells, to produce antibodies specific to those components instead of against a full-fledged virus or bacteria. This then triggers an immune response from the body which helps to protect against infection should the virus or bacteria enter the body in future.

In addition, cytokines are also produced when a subunit vaccine is administered. These proteins serve as messengers between cells of the immune system and help to regulate its response to infection or inflammation. Cytokines play an important role in helping to activate other cells of the immune system which are essential for mounting a defense against infection.

3. Toxoid Vaccines

Toxoid vaccines are created from toxins produced by the pathogen which have been rendered harmless. These toxins, known as exotoxins, are isolated and combined with other substances to create a vaccine that stimulates an immune response in the recipient. The body then recognizes these exotoxins and creates antibodies against them, eventually providing immunity against more infectious forms of the same virus or bacteria. Toxoid vaccines are generally safe and effective but may not provide as strong an immune response as live attenuated vaccines. These types of vaccines are typically used to protect against diseases such as diphtheria, tetanus and pertussis.

What Is The Chemical Reaction That Occurs In The Immune System?

When a toxoid vaccine is administered to an individual, the body's immune system recognizes the exotoxins found in the vaccine and produces antibodies specific to those toxins. These antibodies attach themselves onto white blood cells, such as macrophages and neutrophils, and help to fight off any potential infections.

Furthermore, cytokines are also produced when a toxoid vaccine is administered. These proteins act as messengers between cells of the immune system and help to regulate its response to infection or inflammation.

main types of vaccines, there are also recombinant vector vaccines and conjugate vaccines. Recombinant vector vaccines are made from a live microorganism that has been genetically engineered to express an antigen from another organism; this type of vaccine is used to vaccinate against hepatitis B. Conjugate vaccines are made by linking antigens from different organisms to each other; they are used to increase the effectiveness of vaccines against certain bacteria, such as Haemophilus influenzae type B (Hib).

Vaccines can also be divided into two categories: prophylactic and therapeutic. Prophylactic vaccines are designed to prevent disease by stimulating the body's immune system to produce antibodies; they are used to protect against infectious diseases. Therapeutic vaccines, on the other hand, are designed to treat existing diseases by stimulating the body's immune system in a different way. Examples of therapeutic vaccines include those used to treat cancer and HIV/AIDS.

Immunotherapy

Immunotherapy is a type of medical treatment that helps the body's own immune system fight

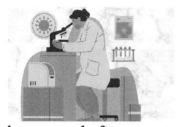

disease. It works by boosting the natural defenses of the body to recognize and then attack cancer cells. Immunotherapy has been used for many years to treat certain types of cancer, but recently more types are being treated with this therapy. Immunotherapy can be used alone or in combination with other treatments such as chemotherapy, radiation therapy or surgery. It is important to note that it does not always work for everyone and some people experience side effects. However, it is an exciting new way to treat cancer and can offer hope to many individuals facing the disease. Immunotherapies are typically used to target tumors in specific areas of the body, but they can also be used to boost the overall health of the immune system. This can allow it to fight off other infections and diseases that could otherwise cause harm. People need to understand that immunotherapy is not a cure for cancer, but can help individuals manage or even beat it.

What Are The Advantages And Disadvantages Of Immunotherapy?

Immunotherapy has become increasingly popular in recent years as a way to fight cancer. This type of therapy offers many advantages, such as being able to target specific tumors without harming healthy cells, as well as being able to boost the overall health of the immune system. It also has fewer side effects than other types of cancer treatment, such as chemotherapy and radiation therapy. However, there are some disadvantages to immunotherapy as well. For instance, the cost can be prohibitive for many people, and not everyone will respond positively to it. Additionally, it can take a long time before any benefits are seen from the treatment.

Immunotherapy can be a very effective way to fight cancer, and it offers many advantages. However, before beginning any course of treatment it is important to discuss all available options with your doctor in order to make the best decision for each individual's situation. Additionally, it is important to monitor one's overall health while undergoing immunotherapy, as there are potential risks, such as an adverse reaction to the treatment or a decrease in the effectiveness of the therapy. With proper care and monitoring, immunotherapy can be an effective cancer treatment.

What Are The Types Of Immunotherapies?

Several types of immunotherapies are used to treat cancer. These therapies work by boosting the body's own immune system to recognize and attack cancer cells. Common examples of immunotherapies include checkpoint inhibitors, CAR-T cell therapy, monoclonal antibodies, and cytokine therapies. Each type works differently to target either specific tumors or the overall health of the body's immune system. It is important to discuss with your doctor which type may be right for you.

Checkpoint Inhibitors

Checkpoint inhibitors are a type of immunotherapy that helps the immune system recognize and attack cancer cells. This type of therapy works by blocking certain proteins in cancer cells, which are called checkpoints. By blocking these checkpoints, the body's own immune system can more easily identify and eliminate cancerous cells. Checkpoint inhibitors have been used to treat several types of cancers, including lung cancer, melanoma, and bladder cancer.

Car-T Cell Therapy

CAR-T cell therapy is a type of immunotherapy that uses genetically engineered immune cells to recognize and attack cancer cells. The immune cells are taken from the patient's blood and modified to identify and target the cancerous cells. This type of treatment has been used to treat certain types of leukaemia and lymphoma.

Monoclonal Antibodies

Monoclonal antibodies are a type of immunotherapy that helps the body's own immune system recognize and attack cancer cells.

This type of therapy works by targeting specific proteins in cancer cells, which are called antigens. When the body recognizes these antigens, it can then eliminate the cancer cells. Monoclonal antibodies have been used to treat several types of cancers, including breast cancer and colorectal cancer.

Cytokine Therapy

Cytokine therapy is a type of immunotherapy that helps the body's own immune system recognize and attack cancer cells. This type of therapy works by introducing cytokines, which are molecules that can activate the immune system, into a patient's bloodstream. When the body recognizes these cytokines, it can then more effectively target and eliminate cancer cells. Cytokine therapy has been used to treat certain types of cancers, including lymphoma and leukaemia.

Immunotherapy is an exciting new way to fight cancer and can be a powerful tool to help individuals manage or even beat the disease. People need to understand all of the risks and benefits associated with any type of treatment before beginning, as well as monitor their overall health during treatment. Additionally, immunotherapy is not a one-size-fits-all solution, and it may not work in every situation.

Immunology's Role In Cancer Treatment

Cancer is one of the leading causes of death

worldwide. Immunology, the study of the body's immune system, can help provide insight into how to best combat cancer in patients. With advances in immunological research, doctors and researchers are better able to understand which treatments will work best for specific types of cancer.

Recent studies have shown that the immune system plays a crucial role in cancer therapy. By stimulating the body's natural ability to recognize and attack cancer cells, immunotherapy has become an important tool for fighting cancer. Immunotherapy can be used to target specific types of tumors by boosting the immune system's recognition of them. Additionally, immunotherapy may also help reduce adverse side effects associated with chemotherapy and radiation treatments.

The ability of the immune system to recognize and fight cancer cells is dependent on a variety of factors, such as genetic makeup, age, and lifestyle. As researchers continue to study immunology's role in cancer treatment, they will be better able to develop more tailored treatments that are effective for each individual patient.

Immunologists are also exploring ways to manipulate the immune system to create an environment that is more conducive to cancer treatment. For example, they are studying ways to stimulate the production of white blood cells, which help fight off infection and disease. Additionally, immunologists are researching how to prevent tumor growth by targeting factors in the body that cause cancer cells to spread.

Immunology's role in cancer treatment has been invaluable in helping to improve the quality of life for cancer patients across the globe. By continuing to research and develop immunology-based treatments, doctors and researchers can help create more effective therapies that are tailored to the individual needs of their patients. With further advances in immunological research, we can all work towards a future where cancer is no longer a threat.

In addition to immunotherapy, researchers are also exploring other methods of cancer treatment such as gene therapy. This approach involves inserting genes into the body that can help fight off cancer cells and prevent their growth. Gene therapy is currently used in some clinical trials for certain types of cancer, though it has yet to be widely accepted as a standard treatment option. As research continues, gene therapy may become a viable option for many types of cancer in the future.

The field of immunology is ever-evolving and researchers are constantly finding new ways to leverage the body's natural defense system against cancer. With continued research and development, we can all work together towards improved treatments that can help improve the lives of cancer patients everywhere.

Immune System's Defense Against Cancer Cells

The immune system is constantly on guard and ready to protect the body from viral, bacterial and other pathogenic threats. This defense also works to identify and eliminate cancer cells. The body's first line of defense against cancer is the innate immune system, which includes macrophages, dendritic cells and natural killer cells.

Macrophages are one of the most important immune cells in cancer defense. They are able to recognize and engulf foreign substances, such as cancer cells, which allows them to remove these harmful invaders from the body. Dendritic cells detect abnormal activity in the body and alert other types of immune cells to respond accordingly. Natural killer (NK) cells also help kill cancer cells by recognizing and targeting specific cell surface proteins.

The adaptive immune system is also an important part of the body's defense against cancer cells. This branch of the immune system uses antibodies to recognize and identify cancer cells, which then triggers a response from other types of immune cells. These responses can involve engulfing and destroying the cancer cells, as well as signaling for additional help from other parts of the innate and adaptive immune systems.

By leveraging the body's natural defense system, researchers can develop therapies that are tailored to each individual patient and their specific cancer type. This knowledge will help inform more effective treatments for cancer in the future.

CONCLUSION

The immune system is a complex network of cells and tissues that helps protect us from infection and disease. It is made up of the innate and adaptive immune systems, which work together to recognize and respond quickly to various threats. The immune system also plays a role in tissue regeneration, controlling our body's internal environment, and responding to tissue grafts and foreign proteins.

The immune system is responsible for protecting the body from foreign particles and organisms. It is made up of a complex network of organs, cells, and proteins that work together to detect intruders and respond accordingly. The body uses a variety of tools, such as antibodies, T-cells, and cytokines to identify foreign invaders. Once an invader is identified, the immune system responds by activating a series of responses designed to eliminate the threat. The response can vary depending on the type of invader and can range from producing antibodies to launching an attack with T-cells. The complexity and efficiency of the immune system is essential for keeping us healthy.

Innate Immunity is a powerful system that helps protect the body from infection. It involves physical and chemical mechanisms that work together to prevent pathogens from entering the body or spreading too far. In addition, it also helps the body recognize foreign particles and distinguish between friend and foe, helping to ensure that the body is only reacting to potential threats. Overall, Innate Immunity is an essential part of our health and well-being and without it, we would be much more vulnerable to infection.

By understanding how the innate immune system works, we can become better equipped to protect ourselves from potential illnesses or infections. Taking steps such as eating a healthy diet, exercising regularly, and getting enough sleep can all help to support a strong and functional immune system. That way, you can be prepared for any potential threats that may come your way.

Functions of the immune system

1. **Pathogen recognition and response**: The primary function of the immune system is to identify and respond to "non-self" — foreign substances, including pathogenic microorganisms that have gained entry into the body. To accomplish this, the immune system utilizes a network of specialized cells and organs that detect pathogens before they can cause an infection. Pathogens are recognized by the immune system via a repertoire of specialized proteins known as toll-like receptors (TLRs).

2. Protection from infection: Once the pathogen or non-self antigen is detected, the body initiates an immune response to protect itself from further damage. This includes the production of antibodies that bind to and neutralize antigens, the activation of complement proteins that can enhance antibody function, and the production of cytokines that act as messengers to coordinate the different parts of the immune system.

3. Immune memory: The body's ability to remember previous encounters with pathogens is an important aspect of the immune response. This process, known as immunological memory, allows the body to respond more quickly and effectively against a given pathogen in subsequent exposures. This is the basis of immunity conferred by vaccines and natural infection.

4. Tolerance: In addition to protecting from infection, the immune system must also be able to distinguish between self and non-self cells and respond appropriately. The body's ability to recognize its own cells as "self" and not mount an immune response against them is known as tolerance. This is essential for the normal functioning of the body, and any disruption to this process can lead to

autoimmune diseases in which the body attacks its own tissues.

5. Homeostasis: The immune system also plays a role in maintaining homeostasis, or balance, within the body. It does this by recognizing and responding to changes in temperature, pH, osmolarity, and other physiological parameters. In addition, the immune system is involved in wound healing, regulation of metabolic processes, and the maintenance of gut microbiota.

6. Metabolic functions: The immune system also plays an important role in metabolism by regulating energy expenditure and promoting nutrient absorption. This includes the production of hormones such as leptin and insulin that regulate food intake, synthesis of cholesterol and fatty acids for energy storage, and absorption of vitamins, minerals, and other essential nutrients. In addition, the immune system is involved in the breakdown of complex carbohydrates into simple sugars that can be used by cells for energy production.

7. Developmental functions: The immune system plays a critical role in embryonic development by establishing a balance between cell proliferation and death. In addition, the immune system is involved

in maintaining tissue integrity and
organization during development and in
controlling inflammatory responses that
are essential for normal growth and
development.

8. Adaptive immunity: The adaptive
immune system is comprised of
specialized cells such as T cells and B cells
that are capable of recognizing foreign
antigens and mounting an appropriate
response. This involves the recognition of
specific antigens by the T cells and B cells,
activation of these cells into effector cells
that produce antibodies, and memory
cells that can respond more quickly and
effectively in subsequent exposures.

9. Innate immunity: The innate immune
system is comprised of a network
of specialized cells and proteins that
recognize pathogen-associated molecular
patterns (PAMPs) on invading pathogens.
This system is the first line of defense
against infection and can respond quickly,
but is less specific than the adaptive
immune system. The innate immune
system also plays an important role in
recognizing and responding to "non-self"
antigens such as cancer cells.

10. Inflammation: Inflammation is a key
element of the immune response that
serves to remove pathogens, damaged

cells and other debris from the body. This is accomplished by the release of various cytokines which recruit immune cells to the site of infection, stimulate the production of inflammatory molecules, and activate hemostatic processes such as clotting and fibrinolysis. In addition, inflammation is involved in wound healing and tissue repair.

11. Immunological surveillance: The immune system is also responsible for surveying the body for abnormal or cancerous cells. This process, known as immunological surveillance, involves the recognition of tumor-associated antigens by specialized T cells that can then mount an appropriate response and limit tumor growth. In addition to this, the immune system helps maintain tissue integrity and organization by recognizing and responding to damaged cells and initiating repair processes.

12. Immunoprotection: The immune system also aids in the protection of the body from toxic substances and pollutants by recognizing these foreign molecules and mounting an appropriate response. This involves recognition of the toxin by specialized receptors, binding to and neutralizing

the toxin, production of enzymes that can break down toxins, and activation of molecular pathways that can detoxify cells and tissues. This is essential for the body's protection from environmental toxins and pollutants.

The development of immunity against allergies depends on a few key elements. First, exposure to the source of the allergy is necessary in order for the immune system to build up immunity. This can be done in two ways: by introducing small amounts of the allergen over time or through immunotherapy.

Immunotherapy involves regular injections or oral doses of increasing amounts of the allergen over a period of time. This allows the immune system to slowly get used to the allergen and develop an immunity against it.

Another way to build up immunity is by avoiding contact with the allergen altogether, whenever possible. Keeping away from strong allergens such as pollen or pet dander can help reduce symptoms and help build up resistance.

Finally, lifestyle changes such as eating a healthier diet, getting adequate sleep, and exercising regularly can help the body's immune system become stronger and better able to fight off reactions to allergens.

At the end of the day, everyone will have their own

unique approach to building immunity against allergies. But with proper education, precaution and the right steps, you can make significant progress in reducing your allergy symptoms.

MAY I ASK YOU FOR A
SMALL FAVOR?

Before you go, please I need your assistance! In case you like this book, might you be able to please share your opinion on Amazon and compose a legit review? It will take only one moment for you, yet be an extraordinary favour for me. Since I'm not a famous writer and I don't have a large distributing organization supporting me. I read each and every review and hop around with happiness like a little child each time my audience remarks on my books and gives me their fair criticism! ☺. In case you didn't appreciate the book or had an issue with it, kindly get in touch with me via email D.beckology@gmail.com and reveal to me how I can improve it.